Island
NURSES

Island
NURSES

Stories of birth, life and death on
remote Great Barrier Island

Leonie Howie & Adele Robertson

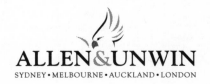

ALLEN&UNWIN
SYDNEY·MELBOURNE·AUCKLAND·LONDON

Allen & Unwin
Level 3, 228 Queen Street
Auckland 1010, New Zealand
Phone: (64 9) 377 3800

Email: info@allenandunwin.com
Web: www.allenandunwin.co.nz

83 Alexander Street
Crows Nest NSW 2065, Australia
Phone: (61 2) 8425 0100

A catalogue record for this book is available
from the National Library of New Zealand

ISBN 978 1 877505 84 3

Internal design by Kate Barraclough
Map by Janet Hunt
Set in 12/17 pt Adobe Garamond Pro
Printed and bound in Australia by Griffin Press

10 9 8 7 6 5 4 3 2 1

Cover photograph captions (clockwise from top left): Leonie in 1973; Adele in 1970; Sunset on Great Barrier Island Aotea

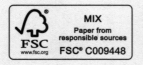

MIX
Paper from
responsible sources
FSC® C009448

The paper in this book is FSC® certified.
FSC® promotes environmentally responsible,
socially beneficial and economically viable
management of the world's forests.

CONTENTS

AOTEA
GREAT BARRIER ISLAND

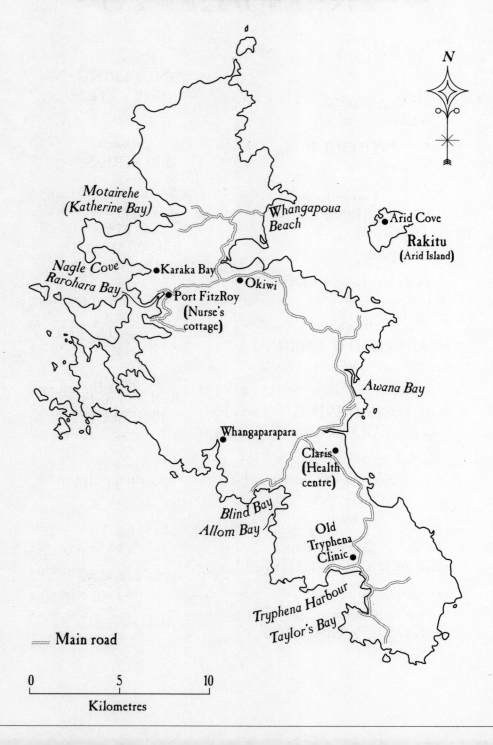

N

Motairehe (Katherine Bay)

Whangapoua Beach

● *Arid Cove*
Rakitu *(Arid Island)*

Nagle Cove
Rarohara Bay

● Karaka Bay

● *Okiwi*

● Port FitzRoy
(Nurse's cottage)

Awana Bay

● Whangaparapara

Claris ●
(Health centre)

Blind Bay
Allom Bay

Old Tryphena Clinic ●

Tryphena Harbour

Taylor's Bay

----- Main road

| 0 | 5 | 10 |

Kilometres

Authors' note

He tapu te tangata
Ahakoa ko wai
Kōhungahunga mai
Tai noa ki ngā tamariki
Tai pākeke mai
Kaumātua mai
Tīpuna mai
He tapu te tangata

This whakataukī expresses the sacredness of man through the times of infancy, childhood, adulthood, our elders and our ancestors. Life is a continuum. We—Adele and Leonie—hold this sacredness at the heart of our practice as nurses and midwives.

Nursing is about the privilege of being able to share in the joys and sorrows of people's lives and of making a difference. It is empowering people to make decisions about their health, birth and death, and supporting them in their choices.

Nursing is about talking, teaching, touching, smiling and crying. Nursing is caring. Life is sacred.

We live on Aotea, an island that locals call a world of its own. We hope to share with you the specialness of the island people and what it means to be a nurse and midwife living and working in such a remote environment. This book is for all those people who have invited us into their lives.

PROLOGUE

TANGI

I did not meet her
on the bordered path
nor detect her fragrance
in the frolic of violets
and carnations.

She did not stroll riverward
to sun-splash and shadows
to willows trailing garlands
of green pathos.

Death was not hiding in the cold rags
of a broken dirge :
nor could I find her

in the cruel laughter of children,
the curdled whimper of a dog.
But I heard her with the wind
crooning in the hung wires
and caught her beauty by the coffin
muted to a softer pain—
in the calm vigil of hands
in the green-leaved anguish
of the bowed heads
of women.
—*Hone Tuwhare (1977)*

It is about knowing.

That is what the textbooks on rural nursing tell you, and it is true. There are ways of knowing people and places, and there is a special combination of these ways that defines rural nursing. You become part of the place and, in so doing, you become part of its people. You know them, and they know you.

We are separately reflecting on this as we stand here to honour Jill. We are shaded by the tree that arches over the heads of the gathering. Cicadas seethe in its branches, and in the background there is the other ubiquitous sound of the Barrier, the sound of the sea, the gentle slap of wavelets on the sandy shore. The sun is warm, and the heat rises as if in answer from the ground. The prospect from the dappled shade where we stand is the sparkling water of Allom Bay, framed by the bush-clad slopes of the hills. Beyond the entrance to the bay is the broad expanse of Okupu, otherwise known as Blind Bay, and the high land behind the far shore. Other high hills rear behind us. There is a sense, standing here, that we are enfolded by the land.

We all drove to Okupu in our modern vehicles, but then relied upon far more traditional Barrier transport to make the final leg of the journey.

We are standing shoulder to shoulder with a group of people whom we have come to know and deeply admire. An outsider might look at them askance—the men variously unshaven and, by some people's standards, in need of a haircut; the women in colourful attire chosen for its practicality rather than for the way it coordinates, or reveals, or covers. Some of them, men and women, choose to be barefoot, and most of the rest are in jandals or sandals. Insiders—and that now includes us—do not notice details like that, though. And we have learned not to judge this assortment of books by their covers.

Ask one of the men what he does for a living, and he will shrug and say he is a digger driver. It is true, but he also has got a Master's degree in English Literature. There is a mussel farmer who used to be a university lecturer in his former life. And over there is a company director who left school at fifteen.

Children are running about freely. It would look to an outsider as though no one was watching over them, but we know that everyone is keeping an eye. They are island babies: they belong to their parents first and foremost, and to everyone else besides. We helped birth many of these children. We helped birth the parents of more than a few of them. We know their stories, as we know the stories of their families, and we can fit them into the wider story of Aotea—of Great Barrier Island—itself.

We are living a part of that story, even now. Jill is being laid to rest. In some ways, it is the final chapter in her story. But, in another way, it is only really the beginning, as her children are here—tearful at the cruel finality of the death of their mother—and, of course, their story goes on. Jill is part of that story. We are privileged to be part of it, too.

As we listen to the speakers—it is the custom on Aotea to give everyone space to address the gathering—we think about our involvement with Jill and her family, all four generations, down through the years. Adele thinks of the first time she met Jill's father, and of Jill's birth stories, and of how the very day Jill's baby was born, her father died.

Leonie remembers, too, and she feels fresh tears in her eyes. You are supposed to maintain boundaries in nursing, between your professional and your personal life, between patients and friends, between your emotions and your rational self. It is not always possible in the enforced intimacy of rural life, and especially not on an island. We are all called upon to perform different roles for one another in a community such as this: nurse one moment, friend the next. Under these circumstances, the boundaries are fluid and negotiable. The textbooks might not tell you that. But it is true.

Leonie thinks of the lines of Hone Tuwhare's poem 'Tangi' and they ring terribly true. She holds all of her memories of Jill as though in a basket: the happy times, the sad and, finally, the most recent and tragic. If she turns her head she can see the very spot where the haunting resuscitation took place only days before—the last time she was to see Jill.

She listens to the kōrero about her friend and patient, and she knows. It is the special kind of knowing of a rural nurse, as much in the heart as in the head.

Chapter 1

LANDFALL

The word 'isolation' comes from the Latin word for island. Apart from the early years, when we trained and worked in hospital situations, our professional lives have been shaped by isolation. People who come to the island for the first time often tell us that they never realised it was 'so far away'. Te Motu o Aotea is the Māori name for Great Barrier Island—the island of Aotea. In Māori, Aotea translates as 'white cloud', and it is also the name of one of the original waka that came to New Zealand at the time of the great migration. It stands as the largest offshore island from the North Island and provides a natural barrier to the Hauraki Gulf. Captain Cook, taking note of this, named it Great Barrier in 1769, and this name remains in common use today, yet many islanders (or 'Barrierites') prefer Aotea.

On Aotea, we're physically isolated. And, while aircraft technology has somewhat closed the gap and we are only half an hour's flying time from Auckland Hospital, time becomes of the essence in an emergency. It is as though time is a currency that is abruptly devalued when someone's life is ebbing away. The turn-around time for evacuation is extended to at least two hours, which is more than enough time for a serious situation to become severe, even fatal.

And, when we are talking about isolation in the context of Aotea, we don't just mean the physical and psychological distance from the mainland and its secondary health facilities. It is also common for first-time visitors to the island to shake their heads and admit that they didn't realise the island was 'so big', or 'so mountainous'. The residents of Great Barrier Island can even be isolated from one another. There are several main communities, tenuously connected by roads. But there are many people living in bays or gullies or on several outlying islands that are accessible only by sea. Telecommunications have advanced dramatically in recent years, but while the rest of New Zealand—and indeed, most of the rest of the world—takes cell phones for granted, the mountainous terrain of the Barrier means there is patchy coverage at best. There is no reticulated power, water or sewerage; people make their own arrangements for each. Each household is like a little island apart. You get this sense in winter especially, when you navigate the wilderness of land or sea and arrive at the home you are visiting to be welcomed into the warmth where, as often as not, there are children running around and the smell of bread baking in a wood stove. Being welcomed into that human warmth is like reaching a port in a storm. It is like making landfall.

The engine note rises and, with a gentle lurch, the plane begins to roll across the tarmac and down the boat ramp. With a swish, it is afloat and taxiing out on to Waitematā Harbour, living up to its name, which means 'sparkling water'. It is high summer, January 1985.

The Auckland boating fraternity are familiar with the comings and goings of the Sea Bee Air aircraft, so there's no need to wait for clear water. The pilot swings the nose of the plane towards Browns Island and eases the throttle lever forward—Adele and the rest of the passengers can see him do this, as there's no bulkhead between the flight deck and the passenger compartment. The engines roar, and spray begins to hiss past the windows as the plane gathers speed. Everyone aboard thinks of Fred Ladd at this moment, the flamboyant seaplane pilot who pioneered this very seaplane service out of Mechanics Bay, and who became famous for his cry 'A shower of spray and we're away!'

The pilot eases back on the throttle and the vibration and hiss of water abruptly cease. The plane skims down the harbour, seemingly a few centimetres from the surface. The wooden lighthouse on Bean Rock flashes past on the left, and Bastion Point and Ōkahu Bay on the right. By the time it is abreast of St Heliers, the plane is in a shallow climb. The last drops of water creep across the windowpanes and are gone, leaving trails of salt behind them, sparkling in the sunshine. By the time the distinctive crater of Browns Island is passing beneath, the plane has flattened into smooth, level flight. Any turbulence Adele feels is internal. She is leaving her comfort zone—not for the first time, but that does not make it any the less daunting—and venturing into the unknown. She consoles herself with the thought that, if she and Shannon, her husband, survived outback Western Australia for as long as they did, then they are ready for anything.

Beyond Waiheke, the colour of the water changes. It is no longer the blue-green of the inner Hauraki Gulf, mottled with rocks and reefs. The white-fringed Noises are sprinkled beyond Rakino Island like a farewell offering. Then the sea turns Prussian blue, and the swell pattern, given complexity by the northern tip of Coromandel Peninsula and the southern tip of Great Barrier Island, is etched undisturbed across it. Whereas boats lazily drag their wakes to and fro among the islands of the inner Gulf, there are only one or two braving the passage to Aotea. They serve only to emphasise the emptiness of this 100-kilometre stretch of sea. And meanwhile the high, rugged profiles of Coromandel to the right, Little Barrier Island to the left and Great Barrier Island directly ahead impress upon Adele the untamedness of their destination.

After 30 minutes' smooth flying, they are approaching Aotea, the high, western coast indented with its many bays and harbours and with its profusion of rocks and islets off the rugged headlands. Through and over the spine of the heavily wooded mountains, Adele glimpses the white sand of the ocean beaches, fringed with surf. She can't suppress an excited grin.

Kaikōura Island, the guardian of the gateway to Aotea's northern port, passes beneath the plane, and then they rapidly lose altitude as the pilot lines up the still, green waters of Rarohara Bay. There are lots of boats—mostly yachts—moored and at anchor, but the pilot's practised eye identifies the clear stretch of water designated as the seaplane access lane. With another shower of spray and deft manipulation of the engine speed, the plane is back on the water. It rocks gently in the wash of its own landing as it threads a course through the watercraft, and then, with a final squirt of power, it grounds on the pebbly beach below the shop. The pilot kills the engines—the passengers' ears ring in the sudden quiet—walks down the aisle and flings open the door for the passengers to disembark.

There is a small group of people standing on the grass, either waiting to greet passengers or ready to depart on the outgoing flight.

Among them is the nurse, who Adele recognises from a previous visit to the island.

'Hi, Fay. Great flight. It's good to finally get here.'

Fay is a similar age to Adele and she looks relaxed but tired. She helps with Adele's luggage as, all about them, people carry mailbags and crates of milk and bread from the plane to the little store. One or two cars fire up. Doors squeal and bang shut, and one by one the vehicles lurch off and grind their way up the gentle hillside.

'I've just got to pick up my mail from the store, if you don't mind waiting,' Fay says.

'Not at all.' Adele shrugs.

Fay has a quick shuffle through her mail and takes a copy of *The New Zealand Herald*. She introduces Adele to the storekeeper. Adele feels the weight of the storekeeper's appraising gaze as they shake hands.

'Welcome to the Barrier,' he says. 'Anything you need, you know where we are.'

Once outside, Fay and Adele make their way across the road to a two-storey weatherboard building.

'The shortest commute ever!' Adele laughs.

Once they have deposited her bags, Fay takes Adele into the lounge, where there is a family, a small boy and his tired-looking parents. After introductions, Fay checks the boy's temperature and provides advice to his parents about what to do in the event of a recurrence of croup. They offer thanks and set off to return to their boat. Fay gives Adele a tour of the clinic, which does not take long. It is a single room that doubles as office and clinic, and there is a little waiting room, which has a toilet off it.

'He came in last night, and we have been up all night steaming and monitoring him,' Fay explains. 'So if you don't mind, we'll have a bite to eat and then I might try to catch up on a bit of sleep.'

This suits Adele just fine. She was up until the early hours helping her husband, Shannon, get started packing up their house. So at one o'clock in the afternoon on her first day at work as the Great Barrier Island public health nurse, Adele finds herself drifting off to sleep in a warm room with a glorious view out over Port FitzRoy and reflecting that this is turning out to be a great job. Fay's exhaustion doesn't strike her as significant—for now, at least.

—m—

'Cooking is on this,' says Fay. It is evening, and she is showing Adele the wood stove in the little kitchen. 'It heats the water, too. There's a wetback on it.' Off to the side are two burners and a grill run by gas for use when the fire is not going. 'Lounge . . . This is my bedroom. You've seen yours. This is the bathroom. The water's cold unless you've had the fire going, but it's not too bad in summer. Then you can be pretty grateful for a cold shower.

'Out here—' she leads Adele outside to a door under the house—'is the wash house. The old copper was used for washing before we graduated to a washing machine.'

They go back inside.

'Luckily we get power from the Forest Service generators. They turn off about ten o'clock every night,' Fay explains. 'After that we're on candles. You have to keep a torch handy. If you've got an emergency in the night, you'll need to get the Forest Service to start up the genny for you. You can try ringing, but the telephone operator here at FitzRoy is hard to wake up. Remind me to tell you about the phones. So, you can try ringing or radioing the Forest Service mechanic, but probably you'll need to drive around and wake him up. I'll take you to meet the crew later on today. Don't be afraid to ring them as they are really helpful. Oh, and remember to keep your door locked at night.'

Fay sees Adele's face, and laughs.

'Oh, no, no, no! There's nothing like that. Nothing to worry about round here. It's just that in an emergency people panic. If your door's unlocked, they are likely to barge right into your bedroom to haul you out of bed. If the door's locked, at least they'll have to bang on your door and you'll have a chance to get dressed first. What I do is keep a change of clothes laid out beside my bed so that I don't have to fluff around in the dark. Once—must have been a bit more tired than usual—we had a bit of a drama and I threw on my clothes and it wasn't until much later on that I realised my dress was on inside out and I'd forgotten to put any undies on! Can you believe that?'

There is a note of uncertainty in Adele's laugh.

'Adele, this is Gwen. Gwen, Adele's going to be the new nurse. You and Myrtle will look after her, won't you?'

'Pleased to meet you.' Gwen beams.

'Gwen and her mum have been wonderful to me,' Fay says. 'You'll see. I don't know what I would have done without them at times. They're always here if you need a cup of tea or someone to talk to. Also, Gwen can help you out with the wood stove, as it's not as simple to operate as it looks.'

Gwen and Myrtle live on the main road at Okiwi. Myrtle keeps a little book in which she has written the names of all the nurses who have worked on the island, complete with the dates they arrived and departed. There's a sort of a family tradition of taking the nurse under their wing.

'My husband was third generation on the island,' Myrtle tells Adele proudly. Myrtle is elderly, but still sharp.

Gwen says, 'When I was a child, Mrs McLean was the nurse. She went on regular trips round the island, visiting people, and she used to stay with us whenever she came past. You even remember her horse's name, don't you, Mum?'

'Tomi.' Myrtle nods. 'His name was Tomi. Of course I remember! Mrs McLean gave Tomi to me when she left the island. No cars in those days. So she used to ride Tomi all around the place. Her trip took a week or more to get to Tryphena and back again, and she had to open more than twenty gates on the way. Off the horse, open the gate, lead him through, close the gate, back on the horse. Twenty times! You don't know how good you've got it these days!'

'The phones!' Fay exclaims. 'I nearly forgot. Good thing you reminded me. Most people are on a party line, which means there could be up to ten other people all connected, each with their own ring tone. We are fortunate to have our own line. When you're going to make a call all you do is crank the handle with one long twist. The whole system only works during the day so that the operator can get a bit of peace at night. But if it's an emergency you do five longs and wait. If he doesn't wake up, you can go across the road to the phone box. Make sure you take a torch, because there are no lights and it's really dark in there. The phone box is switched over to Auckland, so as soon as you pick it up they'll answer. They think you're phoning from overseas, so they'll say, "New Zealand here." Just tell them you're calling from the Barrier. They can connect you to anyone else you want, other exchanges on the island—if they wake up—or on the mainland.'

Adele is nodding slowly, trying to absorb all this.

'Of course, lots of people don't have phones, so the only way to get in touch with them, or for them to get in touch with you, is by CB radio—you know, Citizen Band. We keep the radio on all the time. I'll show you how to use it—nothing to it, really. But remember, everyone can hear you. And don't go presuming that you're the only person on the telephone line, either. In wet weather, the lines can cross, meaning that other people might be able to hear your conversation—interesting for them, especially if they know it's an emergency. On the radio it can be quite good, people listening in. All sorts of people pipe up and say they can help. But not good for patient confidentiality! There is a tongue-in-cheek saying that everyone knows everyone else's business out here, and if they don't they tend to make it up.'

This is the way it goes for the first week. It is hot, and the mānuka and ferns crowding the roadside are heavy with grey road dust. Fay and Adele go for long drives, the red Toyota Land Cruiser rattling and crashing on the corrugated and potholed dirt roads.

Fay introduces Adele to the locals and generally tries to show her the ropes. The detail seems overwhelming, but as time goes by Adele will come to appreciate just how hard it is to give another person a feel for the way of life that rural nursing is—the complex intertwining of your life with those in the community of which you are a part. Add to that the challenges of this particular post—the lack of reticulated power and water, the poor state of the roads, the even worse state of telecommunications—and you find you are treading a fine line between imparting useful information and sending your prospective colleague running for the hills.

The public health nurse at Port FitzRoy is not completely without professional nursing support on the island. Nancy Cawthorn is the part-time emergency nurse at the southern end of the island, and on the third or fourth day Fay introduces Adele to Nancy. Adele is heartened to have such a warm, supportive colleague to call upon if she needs her.

She knows there is a general practitioner on the island, too, and that he holds a clinic once a week at the nurse's cottage in the north, but her employers have made it plain that, as he is in the 'private system', she is not to give him any assistance, nor is he to use any of her supplies. She asks Fay and Nancy about him.

'Oh, Ivan's great,' Nancy says. 'I have a lot to do with him— probably more than we're supposed to, but things out here don't always work the way Auckland thinks they do. Never mind the rules. Ivan's there if you need him.'

At the end of the week, it is time for Fay to leave. She hands Adele a bunch of keys—the vehicle, the clinic and the cottage.

'Keys to the kingdom,' she says, a hint of something like regret in her voice. She squares her shoulders, gives Adele a hug, wishes her well and reminds her that she is only a phone call away (if the telephone works).

'You'll be fine,' she says. 'Just remember—' She stops herself and laughs. If there's anything she has not told Adele by now, it's all a bit late. And, in the end, everyone coming to a rural nursing post has to find out much of it for themselves.

Once Fay has gone, Adele spends the afternoon going through the clinic, looking at paperwork and familiarising herself with the supplies. A sheet of paper in the unruly pile of papers catches her eye. It is entitled: 'Safe Fish Hook Removal'.

That could come in handy, Adele reflects, and puts it in the growing pile of things she will read later. Also among the papers, she finds carbon-copied books of correspondence between head office in Auckland and the nurses who have preceded her in the last twenty years or so. This correspondence makes for interesting reading. It's a litany of complaints about failing machinery, inadequate equipment, and supplies that have gone astray, being dropped at the wrong wharf or simply the wrong island. One makes Adele smile. The nurse asks after the parts she needs to repair her lawnmower. If they don't arrive soon, she says, she will need to buy a machete to get from her door to her car. The replies from Auckland, while polite, seem unsympathetic, and, reading between the lines, Adele can sense the exasperation the island nurses are feeling dealing with the distant government department.

Two weeks after Fay leaves, Myrtle suffers a stroke. She is profoundly affected. Adele, Nancy and Gwen try to put in place a plan to care for her on the island, but it soon becomes plain that it is impractical. Myrtle is flown out to the mainland. It is a terrible thing both for Gwen and for Myrtle, leaving the island on which she has lived her whole life. She does not return, and does not survive long away from Aotea.

There is a knock on the door. Adele opens it and finds no one there. Even as she is peering round the frame to see if she can see who has knocked, there is a thumping at another of the four doors. Eventually, both Adele and the knocker meet at the same door. He is a solid man in a stained singlet and shorts, smelling strongly of fish.

'Good,' he says. 'You are here. My mate has a fish hook in his hand. He's down at the shop looking for you. I'll go get him.'

While he is across the road, Adele frantically searches among the papers on the desk in the clinic. She finds the article on fish hook removal and scans it quickly. The level of technical detail is baffling and unhelpful, so she tosses the paper aside.

The patient and his mate arrive. The barb of the hook is deeply embedded in a finger of the man's left hand.

'I suppose you get a lot of these,' the patient says, to cover up his nervousness.

Adele nods and smiles what she hopes is a competent and confidence-inspiring smile.

Step one, she thinks: make the area numb, so that no matter what you do, it will not be painful.

Once she has administered a local anaesthetic, she considers how to extract the hook. She supposes the trick is much the same as removing a hook from a fish's mouth—push laterally away from the barb and sort of flick it out of the wound in one swift motion. She looks in the cupboard and finds a pair of unusually sturdy-looking surgical pliers. She is immediately grateful, because they have an important, purposeful look about them, which will help bolster the patient's confidence. She grasps the shank of the hook and performs the flicking manoeuvre, familiar from half a lifetime of fishing expeditions of her own.

'Great,' says the patient, as a small drop of blood wells from the wound. 'Lucky we struck someone who knows what they're doing!'

Adele smiles, and both men go off happily to resume their fishing.

Thirty years later, she still has no idea what the proper function of those pliers is. It hardly matters: they have been her tried and trusted fish hook removal tool ever since that day.

———m———

After she has been on the island for six weeks, Shannon arrives, and it is immediately apparent that things are not going to be easy. They both wanted to return to live in a rural area near the sea, and figured some sort of employment would come along eventually, but it doesn't happen immediately. He is used to working, so he sets up a small workshop in the garage at the back of the nurse's cottage. All their married life they have had two incomes, and he struggles with Adele suddenly becoming the main income earner. Once his boat arrives from the mainland, he enjoys having the opportunity to fish and dive on a regular basis. The first time someone says, 'Ah, you're the new nurse's husband,' he takes it quite well. The second time, not so well, nor all the times after that. Adele, meanwhile, tries hard to keep a straight face, thinking of the generations of women who have been assured that they existed only in relation to their husband.

———m———

'Don't worry,' Adele hears Shannon say. 'She'll lie down soon and go to sleep.'

She realises their house guest, a family friend, has been watching aghast as she has burst through the door, dragged the vacuum cleaner out of the cupboard and started maniacally vacuuming the house. Shannon is used to this kind of carry-on after she has come in from an emergency call-out. He has stopped worrying about it.

Adele, on the other hand, *has* been worrying about it, to the point where she even asked Nancy whether she used to experience the same massive surge of adrenaline that Adele gets every time she is called to an emergency.

'Yes, at first I did,' Nancy had replied. 'But not anymore.'

'How long did it take to get past it?' Adele asked.

Nancy shrugged. 'I can't really remember, to tell the truth. But don't worry. It will happen.'

Adele is an experienced public health nurse and midwife, and is skilled at the routine of working with families in these roles. However, she is less experienced or confident about emergency work. She has attempted to remedy this shortcoming by travelling over to Auckland for the occasional afternoon shift in the Emergency Department at Auckland Hospital, as well as a few shifts with St John ambulance. This has helped, but neither the work—nothing quite like the assortment of scenarios that might strike on Great Barrier Island arise in an urban environment—nor the approach can fully equip her for what she is already beginning to experience. After all, the St John staff have the comfort of knowing they have a fully equipped, modern hospital only a few minutes' drive away from the scene of their emergency, and the staff at Emergency have state-of-the-art equipment at their disposal. In the northern part of Great Barrier Island, Adele is both first responder and primary health professional combined. Only in a serious emergency would she call for a patient to be airlifted out, and even then it would take an hour or more for the plane or helicopter to arrive, and the same to get back to the mainland—and that is if weather conditions would let them get off the ground at all.

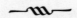

Summer is a frantic time on the Barrier. By 1986 the permanent population has risen to 858, but in summer an armada of private yachts and launches arrive, along with holidaymakers on the planes and the ferries. The population can increase tenfold. This means the nurse's cottage, in the north, is under siege day and night. People present with a range of injuries, ailments and afflictions ranging from the minor—sprains and stings and sunburn—to the more serious—broken bones, suspected heart trouble, respiratory and other infections. Others have forgetfully left their medications at home and imagine they will be able to get a prescription filled on the island, not realising that there is no pharmacy on the island.

It is not just the nature of the work. Adele and Shannon find themselves living in a fishbowl: people are constantly knocking on the doors of the clinic, and their own home becomes a kind of outpatient's ward, where people are being monitored overnight or are awaiting transport off the island. Despite being well served with the quantity of doors—there are four—the clinic does not have a single door that will admit a stretcher or wheelchair, so occasionally patients lie on a stretcher outside while awaiting to transfer to hospital.

The relentlessness of being on-call 24 hours, seven days a week takes its toll. Added to this is the isolation from peer support—Nancy is an hour away at the southern end of the island—and the fact that some of her supervisors in the Public Health Nursing Department are apparently oblivious to the demands and challenges of island nursing. Adele soon realises they have no idea what it is like. On a clear day, you can see Aotea from Auckland. But, as the locals say, it is a world of its own.

Reading the stories of the nurses who have gone before, she notices that after Phyllis Wharfe, the ninth public health nurse on Great Barrier Island who served for five years in the 1950s, no one has lasted in the post for more than two years. Whether this is due to the personal choice of the women involved or to a Health Department policy, Adele can't quite tell. She notices that some were even sent from the mainland to Aotea to recover from stress or illness—a testament, if ever there was one, to how completely the Health Department bureaucracy failed to understand what the life of an Aotea nurse was like.

After Adele has been on the island for a couple of years, she receives a visit from a woman who tells her she was a nurse on the island for a while in the 1960s. She is visiting on a yacht, and would love a bath. Adele is happy to oblige, and keen to hear her story.

Well, the woman says, there had been a series of incidents over several days, culminating in the birth of a premature baby and a man with a serious laceration requiring urgent attention. For some reason—probably bad weather—the plane couldn't come and she had boarded a fishing boat with both patients to rendezvous with a Navy vessel in the Hauraki Gulf. The sea was rough and the transfer was difficult. Once the patients were handed over, she returned with the fishing boat to another harbour further down the island. The skipper of the fishing boat and his family tried to persuade her to stay the night, but, charged with adrenaline, she insisted on walking the forest road home. It is an arduous, up-and-down trek— four or five hours at the best of times. This was late in the day, after a series of long, hard days. Not far down the track, her footwear broke but, undaunted, she pressed on barefoot. Then it started to get dark. She was without a torch, and the depth of Great Barrier Island darkness has to be experienced to be believed. She cut her foot on a sharp stick on the track. By this time, the adrenaline had faded and fatigue had set in. As she walked, the wound on her foot became packed with dirt, and her certainty grew that she had contracted tetanus. By the time she reached Port FitzRoy and saw a house, she was quite distraught. The family who opened the door to this distressed, bedraggled, barefoot, muddy and bloodstained woman were thoroughly taken aback, and wasted no time in calling Auckland. A plane was sent to collect her the very next day.

Adele feels for this nurse, as she can completely understand how such a thing might happen. Challenging situations, plus the exhaustion and sheer physicality of the work on the island, can lead to what Adele now calls 'mini-meltdowns'. Whereas Adele is fortunate to have an understanding husband to support her through difficult moments, she is aware that many before her, just like this nurse, have been on their own.

One day, when she is visiting Gwen, Gwen puts down her cup of tea and picks up what Adele recognises as Myrtle's little book of Aotea nurses.

'Look,' says Gwen.

There, in Myrtle's shaky handwriting, is Adele's name, with the date of her arrival and a dash followed by a blank space. Adele looks at that space and wonders what date will one day be written there.

Chapter 2

ON CALL, ON EDGE

These days, health and safety and risk minimisation are a kind of mantra in most areas of life, not least emergency medicine. St John teaches its trainees that for those attending an emergency, safety at the scene is your first consideration. In Adele's early days on Great Barrier Island, the island's doctor and nurses were usually the scene coordinators as well as the first responders and, in the often isolated scenes of an emergency, not much in the way of extra manpower was always available. However, as long as locals were present situations that initially seemed tricky and insurmountable were generally solved in a practical way. We have faced the same difficulties throughout our career practising on the island, and we still occasionally face them today.

Still, some of the stories of how intrepid the early nurses were put anything we have had to face into the shade. When Adele first told her sister that she was taking up a post on the Barrier, her sister looked concerned.

'You're brave,' she said. 'I heard a story that one of the nurses out there had to visit a patient on an island and, because the boat couldn't land, she had to strip off and swim ashore!'

Adele snorted.

But after she had been on the Barrier for a number of years, she told this story to a group of locals, expecting them to laugh. Instead, they nodded.

'Yes, that was Mrs Mence,' one said. 'She was the nurse here back in the seventies. She received a call via radio link one day to say the caretaker on Rakitu Island—an older man living by himself— had badly injured his back. The hospital wouldn't approve a helicopter evacuation unless he'd been seen by the nurse, so Mrs Mence boarded a boat on the eastern side of the island at Whangapoua Beach. You can only land at Arid Cove, and that day it was pretty rough, with the wind blowing surf on to the beach, and the only dinghy ashore was damaged. So she did the decent thing and stripped down to her underwear and swam ashore. Nancy was a good swimmer, but it still would have been taxing as it was a long way and the middle of winter.'

'What happened to the patient?' Adele asked.

'Oh, we fixed the dinghy while she was seeing him, then we took them back to Port FitzRoy, where Nancy called for a helicopter to come get him later that day. He was able to return to the island a few weeks later.'

We hear these stories from time to time where, in the challenging environment of Great Barrier Island, needs sometimes must.

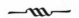

The call comes at midnight. It is the manager of a lodge across the bay and he is reporting an accident—a vehicle off the road. Adele drives gingerly down the wet clay road as light rain falls. When she decides that the track is marginal even for her four-wheel-drive Land Cruiser, she gets out and walks, slipping and sliding through the mud in her gumboots. The pale boles of kauri trees gleam in the beam of her torch on either side of the track. She can hear screaming.

She sees the flash of another torch. There is the lodge manager who made the phone call, sending the beam of his torch down a 30-metre bank to where the underside of a Land Rover can be seen in the tide. There is a young woman crouched in the water beside the vehicle. The screaming is coming from inside.

'It's a local girl,' the lodge owner says. 'She was driving. She's trapped in there.'

'Anyone else involved?' Adele asks.

'There were two passengers, but they're both fine. One of them got out and climbed up to tell me. That's the other one down there with her.'

Adele is wishing, not for the first time, that she wasn't a nurse on Great Barrier Island.

'Do you want me to try to find a way down for you?' the lodge manager asks.

Adele nods gratefully, and without further ado he sets off down the near-vertical bank. About halfway down, he calls back up.

'Probably best if you go back down the track to the head of the bay. You'll be able to wade around. It's still quite shallow.'

'What's the tide doing?' Adele asks.

'It's on its way in,' he replies from down the bank.

Adele walks back down the track, the rain dripping from the trees. She makes her way to the water's edge and then begins walking around the rocks. The water starts flooding over the top of her gumboots. It feels surreal, because, besides the screaming coming from the Land Rover, there is the sound of music, laughter and the clink of glasses. There are dozens of pleasure boats at anchor further out, and the usual holiday festivities are underway aboard them.

Once she reaches the vehicle, she discovers that, apart from having her lower leg pinned, the young woman seems uninjured. She is panicking, however. Her ankle is pinned somewhere around the top of the door frame—she can't have been wearing a seatbelt—and the water is creeping quietly higher. Adele is more worried about the passenger who is waiting with her, as her teeth are chattering and she looks pale and shocked in the torch beam.

The lodge manager arrives at her side.

'We're going to need help getting her out,' Adele says.

'I'll see who I can round up,' he replies.

'Best take her with you.' Adele indicates the passenger. 'She needs to get warm.'

The lodge manager and the shivering girl slosh away.

'Get me out. Please get me out,' the young woman sobs.

'It's OK. We'll get you out,' Adele soothes her. 'Help is on its way.'

Listening to the carousing going on out in the bay, Adele hopes that whatever help arrives is sober enough to be useful.

She doesn't need to worry on that score. When the lodge manager returns, he has a group of fishermen with him who have been too busy smoking their catch to drink.

'The Forest Service are sending a truck with a winch,' the lodge manager reports. 'And I've phoned your neighbour. He's on his way.'

Adele is pleased, because the mechanic and her neighbour must be two of the few locals who were not at the Boat Club that night.

Headlights can be seen through the trees above. It is the Forest

Service truck, but the mechanic calls down that the strop from his winch isn't going to be long enough to reach. He can't get any closer.

Oil and petrol have been oozing from the vehicle, and Adele is up to her waist in oily water. While it is summer, the water is cold. The young woman has been in the water longer than Adele has: she will be getting hypothermic. They need to act.

'We need to get the weight off her leg somehow,' Adele says.

'We could try lifting it,' the lodge manager suggests. 'What do you think, guys?'

There is a general murmur of assent, so the plan is for the men to position themselves around the vehicle and to lift, while Adele attempts to free the young woman's ankle.

Adele positions herself so that she can grasp the leg as close to the ankle as possible. This entails crouching in the water up to her neck.

'Ready when you are,' she says.

'OK. On three. One. Two. Three!'

There is the sound of exertion. The vehicle moves and Adele gently pulls the young woman's leg upward. The young woman screams, and points of light wheel across Adele's vision. She is briefly afraid she is going to faint, but at that moment the leg comes free and the woman floats out of the cab. The men let go of the vehicle, which thumps back into the water.

One of the men carries the relieved young woman to his vehicle as Adele walks beside them.

'I'll drive you to the nurse's cottage so you can look after her on the way,' he says. 'We'll get your vehicle back to you tomorrow.'

The following morning, the girl who climbed up the bank to raise the alarm presents herself to the nurse's cottage. She has a bad laceration on her lower leg that should have been attended to the previous night. Adele has a habit of going over and over every incident and working out what she would do differently next time. She should, she tells herself, have checked both passengers over the previous night. But, with time, she learns that every situation is unique, and the next one is likely to throw up a completely different set of challenges to be negotiated.

The men in the local community go out at low tide, tip the Land Rover the right way up, tow it back on to terra firma and, after it has been hosed out and had new battery acid, engine oil and petrol tipped in, it fires up again—if not quite as good as new, at least adequately restored.

Adele is not quite so lucky. She writes to the Auckland Hospital Board to inform them that she has ruined an entire set of clothes in attending an emergency and would like to claim reimbursement. Her employers cannot seem to imagine circumstances under which they would be obliged to dip into taxpayers' money to supply a nurse with a full set of clothes. This exchange, Adele reflects ruefully, would not look out of place in the historical correspondence register.

Adele and Shannon have an overnight guest. He is an infant who arrived earlier that evening with his father from one of Aotea's inhabited outlying islands. He presented as very unhappy with a high temperature, ragged breathing and a wet, painful-sounding cough— plainly a respiratory infection. Adele administered paracetamol and antibiotics, whereupon it became a waiting game. The little boy's dad agreed to leave him at the clinic overnight so that Adele could monitor him, and she has spent the night sitting beside him, listening to his breathing and occasionally checking his temperature. A little before dawn, his breathing has noticeably eased and his temperature has dropped into the normal range. Adele decides she can afford to get a couple of hours' sleep.

When he wakes up, the boy is bright and alert and ready for his day. Adele is already dressed in a skirt and T-shirt—it is going to be a scorcher. She has fed the toddler and organised the medications for his family to take back to their isolated home. It is 9 am. There is a knock at the door. A woman is standing there, looking very anxious.

'It's my husband,' she says. 'He's not very well.'

The symptoms she describes are alarming. Adele phones the shop and asks if someone can mind the toddler until his dad arrives. One of the young women races across the road to take over, so Adele slips on a pair of jandals and jumps in the car with the woman. It is only a short drive—50 metres—but the emergency equipment is in the back. The woman indicates a dinghy pulled up on the boat ramp. Adele loads the gear she thinks she will need and they push off. The woman starts the outboard and, after a short ride, they are at the yacht.

Aboard, Adele finds the woman's husband sitting on his bunk, clammy and nauseous and complaining of severe, crushing chest pain that is radiating down his left arm. She wraps the band of the blood-pressure cuff around his upper arm as the sunlight reflected from the water paints patterns on the roof of the boat's cabin.

'Have you ever had heart trouble before?' she asks, and the patient nods. His history and chest pain, together with his blood pressure, which is very high, puts the diagnosis beyond doubt. It is obvious to Adele that he is having a myocardial infarction—a heart attack—and the pain is caused by the death of muscle tissue that is being starved of oxygen by a blockage in a coronary artery. This is a very serious situation. At this time on the island, Adele has only a limited range of drugs; if the man's heart stops, she will have to perform CPR (cardio-pulmonary resuscitation) in a very confined space. The boat has a radio but reception in the harbour is poor, and she has no other means of communicating with Auckland Hospital. High-tech gear, such as a portable defibrillator, and even items that will one day be taken for granted on the island, such as a cell phone or VHF radio, are nothing but a twinkle in some electrical engineer's eye at this point.

Adele has fitted an oxygen mask to the patient's face and is in the process of inserting an intravenous line so that she can administer drugs as efficiently as possible when she hears the seaplane approaching, followed by the characteristic splash and surging roar of the engines as it lands and threads its way through the moored vessels to the beach. The yacht rocks gently in its wash.

Soon afterward, there is the sound of an approaching outboard, which cuts out close to the boat. There is a bump and a series of thumps on the hull. The face of one of the more colourful locals appears in the companionway.

'Ah, there you are, Adele. You right? Mike on the fuelling jetty thought I better check on you, because you'd been gone a while.'

Adele is very pleased to see him. 'I have an emergency,' she says. 'Can you ask the pilot of the seaplane if he can assist me by taking a patient to Auckland, please?'

'Of course,' he says, and disappears. His outboard starts and fades.

'I really need to go to the toilet,' Adele's patient says. She is not keen to let him go, because the toilet is down a couple of stairs in a tiny little cupboard called the head. If his heart failed there, CPR would be an impossibility.

Soon the local is back.

'Plane's right to take him to the mainland. The pilot says he'll come alongside. We can use my boat to get him across.'

(Adele only learns later that he had sped up and grounded his boat next to the seaplane, leaped ashore and yelled authoritatively, 'The nurse is commandeering this plane!' Oh, to have that sort of power, she reflects.)

They are going to have to get the patient on his feet and make him climb in and out of boats. Adele decides that letting him go to the toilet is not much more of a risk. He makes his slow way to the head. There is the intermittent sound of running water, but as minutes pass and he does not reappear she begins to wonder what is keeping him. He is taking ages.

'Are you all right?' she calls.

'Fine,' comes his muffled reply.

When he finally emerges, Adele sees that he has washed his face and combed his hair neatly.

'I feel fine, now,' he announces. 'No pain whatsoever. No need to send me to hospital.'

'Let me check you again,' Adele says. She checks his vital signs. His blood pressure has dropped alarmingly low, and his pulse is rapid and weak.

'You definitely need to go to hospital,' she tells him. 'The reason your pain has gone is that part of your heart muscle has died. You are still at as much risk now as you were when you had the pain.'

It is a difficult exercise getting him off the yacht, into the boat and then on to the seaplane. Adele boards the plane with him and suggests he lie down.

'No.' He waves her away. 'I'm fine. I'll sit like everyone else.'

He is still very pale and unwell-looking. Adele watches him anxiously for the duration of the 30-minute flight. When the plane lands at Mechanics Bay, Adele asks her patient to stay sitting until the ambulance that is waiting can drive over to the plane. But it stays at the gate. She walks over to ask them to come closer, so that he is spared as much exertion as possible, but when she turns around she sees the patient being escorted to the terminal by a couple of Sea Bee Air staff.

She rushes over.

'What going on?' she asks.

'Oh, we're just taking him into the terminal to get a few details.'

'I'm fine,' the patient adds.

'No, really. It's best he comes in the ambulance now,' Adele says firmly. 'I'll give you his details later.'

'I really don't know what all this fuss is about,' the patient protests as he is loaded into the ambulance for the short ride to the hospital. And, when they arrive and there is no wheelchair available, he insists on climbing out and walking under his own steam. In the cool of the air-conditioned hospital, Adele is acutely conscious that she is not wearing a bra. She is surrounded by health professionals—her colleagues—in their neatly pressed white uniforms and here she is, standing in her jandals and dressed in a T-shirt and skirt with her nipples poking out. It is hard to maintain an aura of professionalism under these circumstances. She is feeling pretty rustic. It takes her right back to her days in outback Australia, where she often showed up in the sanitised Emergency Room covered in dust and dirt and with streaks of baby poo on her uniform. Adele is spinning out at this point: she knows she has witnessed a man having a heart attack—he is lucky his heart hasn't stopped—but she is afraid she will not be believed.

Happily though, Auckland Hospital is expecting a cardiac patient, and his insistence that he is perfectly well falls on professionally deaf ears. The nurse lies him down and hooks him up to an electrocardiogram. She watches the trace for a few minutes, and then strides over to a telephone on the wall. The room rapidly fills with personnel and equipment. Adele is happy to step into the background. As the adrenaline fades and the relief washes over her, the long night spent watching over the sick baby begins to catch up with her.

'Look, this is all some kind of mistake,' she hears the patient say as she prepares to take her leave. 'There's nothing wrong with me. Can't I just go home?'

'You are not going anywhere,' the doctor replies shortly. 'You've suffered a major heart attack. You are lucky to be alive. We're admitting you to Coronary Care.'

Eventually, one of the nurses notices Adele and invites her into the staff room for a hot drink. Adele sips her coffee gratefully, but wonders how she will ever summon the courage to ask someone for the loan of enough money to get to the airport. She had not thought to bring a purse or even any money; she is standing in Auckland Hospital exactly as she walked out of the door at Port FitzRoy that morning.

She never does manage to pluck up the nerve. But she remembers that, when she was working at St Helen's Maternity Hospital, she and the other midwives often went by ambulance to Auckland Hospital with women and babies. All they had to do to get home was to present themselves at the orderlies' office and ask for a taxi voucher. So, when she has finished her coffee, she walks along to the office.

'Hi,' she says to the man behind the desk, using her most confident voice. 'I'm the nurse from Great Barrier Island. I have just escorted a patient over and I need a taxi voucher to go to the airport.'

To her delight, bordering on disbelief, he nods and hands over a voucher, just like that, no questions asked. It is a simple matter to get a taxi, then, and once she is at the airport she is on familiar ground. She is confident Great Barrier Airlines will fly her back to the island on promise of payment, and, typically, they go one better: there is no charge at all. By the time the plane lands at the Okiwi aerodrome, Adele is feeling almost cruisy.

Shannon is there to meet her. 'There's good news and bad news,' he says.

'What's the bad news?' she hardly dares to ask.

'The family with the baby left their antibiotics behind.'

Adele groans. It seems this long, long day will never end.

'Don't worry,' Shannon says. 'I've got the boat in the water and we can run them out to the island as soon as we get home.'

'You said something about good news?' Adele asks.

'The good news is that Judith says dinner is cooked at her place. She's not expecting conversation. All you have to do is eat and go home to sleep.'

That is almost how the evening pans out. But at midnight there is a knock at the door.

'This is ridiculous!' mutters Shannon. 'I'll go. They better be dying, otherwise I'm going to tell them they can come back tomorrow!'

Adele listens to the murmured conversation at the door. Shannon reappears.

'You'd better get up,' he says. 'There's blood!'

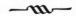

It is not always fraught. There are magical times, too. One hot, sunny autumn day—the sea is like a deep blue mirror—Adele puts on the backpack in which she carries her gear and retrieves the baby bag from the back of her four-wheel-drive. In these early days, most of what she does is home visits. Often the weather is awful and the walking from place to place is arduous, but on days like this . . .

This, she thinks, *is going to be a good day at the office.*

She walks along the sand at the head of Blind Bay to the start of the track, through the bush and over the hill to the next bay, and is spellbound every step of the way by the stillness, the quiet, and the sheer beauty of her surroundings.

Her first call, for a cup of tea and a chat, is to an elderly man with medical problems. He lives in one of two small baches that his family have built and which they occupy during the holidays. Adele admires how well set up he is: outside the little building he has a pile of mānuka logs beside a trestle that he has cunningly designed and constructed to make the job of cutting firewood easier.

'You're pretty isolated here,' Adele says over their cup of tea. 'How do you cope with that?'

'Oh, it's not bad at all. The neighbours are always dropping over. I'm never on my own for long.'

He talks about his wife, now deceased, and about his family on the mainland. He describes his beloved daughter, Jill, who loves the Barrier and comes across whenever she can. He hopes she will join him here soon on holiday.

Adele sets off again along the clay track, up and over a hill to the next bay. As she descends the hill through the bush, she can hear a chainsaw revving. When it falls silent, she hears the sound of chopping instead. Soon the track opens to a fresh clearing. It is the middle of nowhere, but there is a man standing in a drift of reddish sawdust and surrounded by fallen mānuka. He has obviously been working hard for some time. Adele stops for a chat.

'I'm going to build a house here,' he says. He tells her a bit about himself. He has been working for the last little while on prawn trawlers in Australia. He has long had a dream of settling on Great Barrier Island and building his own home.

The track takes Adele away from the coast and into the bush, and she finally reaches a sun-filled house nestled beside a stream surrounded by native bush. The family who live there, far, far from anywhere, welcome her. She has come to see the latest addition—a plump, healthy newborn whom they have only just brought home from the mainland. Adele performs the checks she has come to do. Everything is well, and she walks back to her vehicle for the hour-long drive home.

Over the next few years, she makes this journey—and lots like it—several times. Other babies are born in the meantime, and partly out of consideration for Adele, and partly to turn the well-child checks into a social occasion, mothers and babies gather in a single home for her visit. When she walks this route, she drops in on the elderly man. Eventually his health deteriorates to the point where he has to relocate to be with his family on the mainland. Soon after that, Jill moves into his bach. She will become a firm friend of ours.

The rural nursing experience is tough on Adele and Shannon's relationship in some ways, but there is a silver lining. It is an eye-opener for Shannon. In their previous lives—rural nursing in Australia, working as a midwife in Auckland—Adele has gone off to work in the same way as Shannon has gone off to work. He worked as a workshop supervisor for a Western Australian iron-ore mining company, and in New Zealand he plied his trade as a motor mechanic. His professional life probably had its ups and downs, its dramas and its frustrations, but he did not really feel the need to share them with Adele. Nor did he stop to think that nursing might be different. Consequently, he used to have little idea of how complex and emotionally demanding Adele's job could be. She became used to internalising a lot of the stress and anguish of her nursing.

Great Barrier Island has changed that. He has been in the thick of it, right from the start. One night, Adele sets off to pick Shannon up from the Port FitzRoy Boat Club, the only place resembling a pub in the north of the island. As she drives past the wharf, the beam of her headlights picks out a body lying motionless in the middle of the road. A little further on, she can see a motorbike on its side, its headlamp still illuminated. She stops and climbs out.

'It's Adele, the nurse,' she says to the man. 'Can you hear me?'

'Yes,' he mumbles.

'Are you hurt?' she asks.

'No,' he replies. 'Just want to sleep.'

'Well, you can't stay here,' she says. 'You'd best come to the clinic so I can check you out.'

'No, I'm right, thanks,' he says.

It takes a while, but she finally manages to persuade him that there are better places to lie down than in the middle of the unlit road on a moonless night—especially when everyone else at the Boat Club will be making their own, not necessarily cautious, way home very shortly. Adele helps him up and he limps to the car. By the time they reach the clinic, he is starting to feel pretty sore, and Adele is wondering how she is going to get him inside. But at that moment, Shannon turns up. He had given up on the ride Adele had promised him and decided to walk home. Together, they help the rider into the clinic, where Adele examines him and dresses his cuts and grazes. While there does not appear to be anything seriously wrong, she wants to monitor him for concussion, so she and Shannon help him to settle on a mattress in their lounge. During the night, Adele gets up every hour to check on him.

'Thanks for helping out last night,' Adele says when Shannon emerges the next morning.

'No worries,' Shannon says.

You will hear people in Emergency refer to 'car versus bike' situations, signifying a collision between a car and a motorcycle. Well, one night Adele has a 'cow versus bike' scenario to deal with: she receives an early-evening phone call to say that a cow has stepped into the path of a local man riding home from work. A workmate travelling behind him saw his motorcycle on the road. When he stopped, he found his friend, who had been thrown into a drainage ditch. The cow appeared to be unharmed.

When Adele arrives at the scene, it is obvious that the man has fractured his femur and will need to be evacuated to hospital. She writes instructions on a piece of paper and sends a bystander to the closest telephone exchange to ring for a helicopter. He returns to say it is all organised. Adele now needs to get an intravenous line in, so that she can administer drugs to manage the pain and keep his blood volume up, but it is dark and cold and the man's veins are such that it would be a challenge to get the needle in if she were in the clinic, let alone beside an unlit road. She decides it is best if they take him straight to the airstrip, so that there is no delay for the helicopter transportation.

At the airstrip, they wait what seems an age, but only fifteen minutes have elapsed when someone arrives from the telephone exchange to say that, for some operational reason or another, there will be a considerable delay in the helicopter's arrival time. Adele decides she will transfer to a nearby house that has a generator and good lighting. The patient is taken inside on a stretcher and placed on the floor, where Adele kneels and prepares to insert the intravenous line. At that moment, the door bangs open and a drunk visitor lurches over.

'Outta the way,' he says, trying to push Adele aside. 'I can sort this. I gotta first aid certificate.'

Adele is afraid he will blunder over the broken leg. The patient doesn't look too happy about the proposed change of caregiver, either.

'I've got a first aid certificate, too, as it happens,' Adele says curtly. 'Now go away!'

The other locals who are helping hustle the drunk man out of the room. With the line in, Adele is able to get the pain under control, and soon they hear the throb of the helicopter's rotors. With the man safely installed and the chopper beating its way back to the mainland and Auckland Hospital, she can get to bed.

Adele puts down her book. She could have sworn she heard someone calling out. It is a hot, still night, and she has all the windows of her bedroom in the nurse's cottage open.

There it is again. It definitely sounds like someone calling for help.

Adele dresses and goes outside on to the lawn.

'Help!' a faint voice calls. She cannot see anyone.

'Is someone calling for help?' she shouts.

'Yes! Me! Help!'

'Where are you?' she calls.

'At the wharf,' comes the reply. Adele walks the 50 metres down the road to the wharf where there is a cargo barge tied up. She still can't see a soul.

'Where are you?' she calls.

'Down here.'

She looks over the edge of the wharf and sees the skipper in the tide with his back pressing against the hull of the barge and his feet propped against the wharf.

'Why don't you swim to the ladder?' she asks.

'I can't swim,' he replies.

Adele looks around for something to toss to him, and sees the water hose coiled on its reel. She is just unwinding it when she hears voices up the hill. It seems the crew of the vessel are on their way down from the Boat Club. She drops the end of the hose to the man in the water and tows him to the ladder. He is just gratefully climbing the ladder when his crew arrive along with one of the local women.

'Are you injured?' Adele asks the dripping man.

'Tore my back up a bit on the wharf barnacles,' he replies.

'Let's get you aboard and I'll have a look.'

Just as they are about to step over on to the deck of the boat, one of the crew members, who seems to have surveyed the scene in front of him and jumped to the wrong conclusion, steps forward and begins to abuse Adele.

The local woman leaps to her defence. 'How dare you talk to our nurse like that?'

Adele and the skipper board the boat and go into the galley, where he strips his wet shirt off so that Adele can examine the abrasions on his back. Overhead, the arguing continues between the angry crewman and the staunch local woman. They abruptly cease, and there is a loud splash. She has evidently shoved him off the wharf.

Adele looks from the skipper to another of the crew members who has come down to the galley.

'Should I be worried that there's someone else in the tide?' she asks.

'No,' the skipper says. 'He'll sort himself out.'

The crewman nods. And sure enough, as Adele leaves the boat, the chastened crewman is standing dripping on the wharf.

That was not the first time someone had landed in the tide after a night at the club, either. One time, Adele and Shannon listened as a wife abused her husband, seemingly without drawing breath, for the five minutes it took them to walk to the wharf. They could even hear her voice over the sound of the boat motor once it started, and her husband didn't utter a word the entire time. Suddenly there was a splash, then silence.

Shannon and Adele looked at one other.

'Keep well out of that one,' Shannon said.

A short while later, they heard the boat set off and the woman's voice start up again. It was a relief when they had faded into the night.

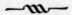

It wasn't only people who went into the water. One evening, one of the locals returned from Auckland with a new set of false teeth and promptly lost them overboard. Replacing them was going to be prohibitively expensive. He was devastated.

On a long shot, Adele and Shannon went down to the wharf at about midnight at dead low tide, and walked around in the mud with a torch.

'Look,' said Shannon.

There, in all their glory, were the teeth, grinning at them.

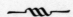

The work, especially in summer, is relentless. The sheer range of emergency situations to which she is called is challenging and stressful. One day, Adele phones her supervisor in Auckland and tells her that she does not think she will be able to stand another summer like it without extra assistance. So for several years, Fay, her predecessor in the job, returns to the island for three weeks each summer. It is never again as busy as that first year.

Chapter 3

PART OF THE FABRIC

Since early European colonisation, Aotea has been subject to discrete 'waves' of settlement, usually determined by the economics of the day. Māori were long established here, of course. They settled mainly around the coastal edges in a number of kāinga (villages), and lived in a kind of symbiosis with the land and its resources. Evidence of these and of pā sites—fortified villages, of which at least 32 have been recorded—can be found. These pā were seasonally occupied from the 1600s by Ngāti Rehua—Ngāti Wai ki Aotea, the present-day tangata whenua of Aotea.

The first Europeans were engaged in 'extraction' industries—whaling, mining for gold, silver and copper, kauri timber and gum-digging. Once these industries had each run their boom and bust course, a new phase in the island's history would begin. Farming eventually became a large industry—twenty settler farms sent a weekly load of cream off to the mainland.

Tangata whenua and the pioneer families remain at the core of the community to this day, as the largest private landowners. They have persisted through many generations and are understandably resourceful and self-reliant, having adapted to the hardships of the Aotea way of life over time.

The next wave of settlement was, for want of a better word, the 'hippies', who were seeking an alternative lifestyle to the mainstream. They set up cooperative communities and sought to be self-sufficient, and had in common with the settler families the same pioneering spirit and self-reliance. They were interested in preserving the environment with which they were interacting. Many of these people and their children still remain.

More recently, there have been those who have deliberately sought out the kind of lifestyle for themselves and their families that only places like Aotea can still provide. Often these are tradespeople and those who work in the service industries, and they have contributed a great deal to the island's infrastructure, bringing skills and a strong work ethic. And, as a constant for very many years, there have been families who own baches on the island. While they do not live on the island year round, they have a long-standing link to and passion for it.

The islanders are largely accepting of difference and diversity. There can, of course, be a range of opinions on any given topic that can erode even the best of relationships. But in times of need the community comes together, and while it is a patchwork rather than a smooth, seamless whole the Barrier community is still a rich piece, stitched together by the shared fact of isolation. In the end, everyone is (almost literally) in the same boat. Above all else, the Great Barrier

Island community is an outstanding example of the way people in isolated communities are resilient and self-reliant and will find a way to make things work. One of the rewards of rural nursing here is that you see first-hand the basic human talent for caring, building and maintaining a strong community network.

And, luckily for us, one of the things that the islanders universally agree upon is the necessity of good healthcare. They care for each other as well as supporting us in our efforts to care for them.

'What's your ETA at the wharf likely to be? Over,' Adele says. She releases the transmit button on the hand-piece of the CB radio. There is a burst of static, and after a short silence the speaker crackles into life.

'Ooh, give us forty-five minutes, I reckon. Over,' the voice replies.

'Roger,' Adele replies. 'Bring him up to the clinic when you arrive. See you then. Nurse's cottage over and out.'

Adele hangs up the hand-piece and walks into the lounge. She sits back down in front of the television, pleased that there will be time to watch the end of the programme she has been enjoying before she needs to deal with the emergency.

Well, look at me, she thinks, amazed. *I am not rushing around checking my emergency gear. I am not all worked up fretting about the procedures I might need to perform. I am not anxious at all!*

It has taken six months of living on adrenaline to reach this point. Six months of feeling the catch in her breath and the race of her pulse with the news of each new drama. But now she has come to realise that the situations are never quite as bad as people report, unless they are actually performing CPR.

For example, she was once told a child had fallen 50 metres down a cliff and was bleeding internally! But when Adele arrived the child was sitting up in bed eating an ice-cream, and it turns out it was more of a roll down a hillside than a plunge from a cliff.

Or a resident overlooking Okiwi airfield phones to say a plane has crashed on take-off! Adele packs everything she thinks might be useful in treating the horrendous trauma she is expecting—fractures, contusions, internal injuries, burns—and, even so, feels she is going to a disaster area with a Band-Aid. It turns out that, although the plane is badly damaged by the forced landing in a farm paddock, the pilot and the local family on board have suffered minor physical injuries. Adele's Band-Aid is sufficient.

Late one night there is a pounding on the door. A panicked local reports that a man who was riding on the tray of their truck on the way back from Claris has fallen off on to the road! 'Hurry,' he says. 'He is bleeding—covered in blood!'

Adele rushes down the stairs and hurries to the roadside in the dark, thinking head injury, major skin loss, embedded gravel, fractured limbs. She can dimly see the man's face. His hair is matted and his skin is pale and covered in dark rivulets. Adele starts to talk to him, anxious to engage him and assess his level of consciousness. To her surprise, he responds quite brightly. She feels for his wrist and locates the pulse. It is strong and steady, not weak and rapid as she expects. Adele flicks on her torch, and plays the beam over him. Everyone starts laughing. He is covered from head to toe not in blood, but in mud. The patient tries to laugh, too, but gasps in pain. It is not all high comedy: he has fractured a few ribs.

The reason Adele coped was the support she was getting—from Shannon, obviously—but also from the community. Gwen became a close friend. While Adele first started visiting her on a regular basis to see how she was coping with the loss of her mum, the boot was soon on the other foot in those sessions. In those early days, she sometimes set off to perform her daily round of home visits but became suddenly overwhelmed with the feeling that she could not go through with them. At moments like those, she would drop in on Gwen. Gwen would just seem to know when she saw Adele's face that all Adele needed to gain composure and perspective was a friendly cup of tea and a laugh.

There are others in Adele's network, too. When she arrived on Aotea, a young mother—one of only two other women of near age in the vicinity—befriended Adele and suggested that she come along to a quilting session with her.

'I don't know the first thing about quilting,' Adele said.

'Doesn't matter,' her new friend said firmly. 'If you can sew, then you can quilt.'

So Adele became a quilter. The venues for the sessions varied. Often Adele had to take a boat to get to the meeting. Other members of the group walked up to an hour through the bush. The food was always outstanding, as everyone brought a dish cooked to their favourite recipe for a shared lunch. But, more importantly, these quilting sessions became a great source of emotional sustenance for Adele. The conversation was always interesting, and there was no pressure to converse. Sometimes she was so tired that she would just sit and absorb the atmosphere. Children ran in and out of the houses: it was an adventure day for them as well, a break from their accustomed isolation, having all these people around. The group worked communally, making quilts for each other as well as for weddings, new babies and as fundraisers. The group made an Aotea quilt as a fundraiser for Greenpeace, and were excited to hear that it was won by a woman whose house had burned down and who had lost everything. Adele always came away from the sessions energised and relaxed. And, even as she sat side by side with other members of her community, stitching together their quilts, she was herself being stitched into the fabric of that community. In a sense, she too was becoming part of an Aotea quilt.

The biggest lack she feels in her early days on the Barrier is the lack of professional support. Her employers in Public Health are Auckland-based and therefore urban. Her first Director of Public Health Nursing was a rural public health nurse in Northland who understood the effects of isolation and the scope of situations that a rural nurse might be called upon to deal with. She also made several visits to the island to see first-hand how Adele was coping. But, since she retired, relations with the new management have become tense and she does not feel safe disclosing to them the anxieties and feelings the work generates. She has been obliged to look elsewhere for strength and support.

She sees Nancy Cawthorn at least once a week and, as she suspected when they first met, Nancy has been a huge help, a fount of wisdom and experience about the unique demands of rural nursing in general, and nursing on Aotea in particular.

In spite of the bureaucratic decree not to have anything to do with Ivan, the GP, it is plain to Adele that they both have the interests of the islanders at heart. She is impressed by Ivan. Unlike many doctors in her experience, he is quite willing to seek help if he is unsure about anything. He possesses the rare ability to instruct—Adele is learning a lot under his tutelage—while also supporting and affirming.

Adele's background is in what is called community nursing. Shannon and she were married shortly before she completed her nursing training. A year after she completed her training, they moved to Australia. Coming from the New Zealand winter, they wanted a warm climate, and they settled on Port Hedland in the Pilbara region of Western Australia. Shannon got a job with a mining company, and Adele at the local hospital. This introduction to Australian Aboriginal people and their culture intrigued her so, in an effort to find out more, she applied for a job in community health. Consequently, what was initially intended to be a six-month stay turned into seven years.

She was given some training. She was put behind the wheel of a long-wheelbase, four-wheel-drive Toyota Land Cruiser and taught how to drive around and around in an abandoned Perth quarry, in order to prepare her for driving in the outback. There was no doubt the vehicle was fit for purpose. But when she was given her first caseload she sat at her desk with a pile of records of the families she was to visit in town that day and she had an anxiety attack. She knew next to nothing about Aboriginal people. She was going into strange territory, all on her own, to knock on the doors of people she had never met and who had never heard of her and who may or may not want her to be there. What would she say? How would she feel if they were rude or hostile? What if the timing was simply wrong for them? What if there were dangerous dogs or drunken or violent people in the house? She was a hospital-trained nurse. Hospital training, she realised, hadn't prepared her for work in the community at all.

She realised that the only way to deal with her fears was to confront them. She made her rounds, and for the most part was very warmly received wherever she went. She found that she needed to learn another way of thinking, talking and operating. Time moves more slowly in the community than it does in the pressure-cooker of a hospital, and it relies intensely upon the building up of relationships and trust. The focus is not on the performance of tasks; rather, it is on a partnership that involves helping people to help themselves over time. It is often less threatening to start on minor issues and build up to the bigger ones, so as not to compromise that fragile trust. The focus is on the person—or, more often, the family—not on a particular problem.

The clinic out of which they were based was little more than an old shed in the grounds of the hospital. There was a tiny waiting room— so small that most patients preferred to sit outside on the grass— and besides that it comprised three rooms: one was a storeroom, another was for the doctor, and the other was for the administrator and nurses. There were six people, but only three desks—reflecting both the low priority health funders gave to Aboriginal health at that time, and the expectation that community nurses would spend most of their time out in the community.

Sure enough, her first week in the job was not over before Adele was directed to do a station visit. She stood in the doorway of the storeroom staring at the shelves of supplies and felt completely overwhelmed.

'I don't know what I'm supposed to do,' she said to the administrator.

'What you do is you fill three of the eskies [as the Australians call chilly bins] with drugs, dressings and vaccines, and you put the eskies, the baby scales, the measuring board and the box of patient notes in your vehicle and you head off.'

Adele hit the road. The vehicle was air-conditioned and had a built-in water tank (for hand-washing) as well as a 12-volt refrigerator for storing vaccines, and a radio link to the office and the Royal Flying Doctor Service base. The outback was another kind of isolation. The empty spaces and the heat; the ragged, parched vegetation extending to the broad, unbroken horizon. It was possible to feel pretty alone out there.

Adele's biggest fear was that she would miss the turnoff from the main road to the station, or that the vehicle would get bogged somewhere along the way. Her heart was in her mouth as she negotiated a riverbed, but once she was across it was plain sailing to the first camp at the station. She had barely got the back door of the vehicle open before an orderly line of mothers and children had formed. Adele wanted to take about ten of the children back to the hospital with her, but the hospital only had eight paediatric beds. How to choose who stayed and who went? So Adele opened the chilly bin containing the medicines and started dispensing. This was the beginning of her lifelong work with women and children.

The area that Adele's service covered was a little over a million and a half acres. There were some mining communities in her territory—the towns of Shay Gap, Goldsworthy and Telfer—but most of her work was in far-flung Aboriginal station communities such as Strelley, Lalla Rookh, Warralong and Yandeyarra.

Adele soon learned that the women she was working with lived in a traditional society where men had all the power and made all the decisions while their wives were regarded as mere chattels. Aboriginal women were doubly condemned—they were treated as second-rate both by their own society because they were women, and by wider Australian society because they were Aboriginal.

As a nurse working with Aboriginal communities, Adele herself was often treated badly by some of the medical and nursing staff of the hospital. She did not fit the 'nurse' stereotype. Instead of appearing pristine in white with tidily groomed hair and make-up on, meekly deferring to the doctors' wishes, she came in after a long clinic day, dusty, sweaty and tired, with patients to be admitted—and it clearly irked the doctors that a nurse would presume to make this decision. Quite often an ill infant would have soiled her uniform. Her appearance was bad enough. As time went by, she learned to be assertive and to demand that her patients be given the treatment and respect they required.

It was hard work, physically certainly, but far more so from a psychological and emotional perspective. Adele's Aboriginal clients died. They were beaten to death by their husbands, they died in prison cells from injuries that should have been treated in hospital—a health worker and his pregnant partner were electrocuted in a shower block that had been wrongfully wired by a council contractor. They died from poverty, alcohol abuse and a lack of adequate and appropriate health services, housing and clean water. Adele had imagined that it would feel good to be making a difference. Instead, she found it soul-destroying to be confronted daily by so much injustice in the face of which she and her clients were all but powerless.

One day, towards the end of her time in the job, she received a note from one of the young mothers she had been caring for.

Dear Sister Dell, it read. *The baby is born. She is called Mary and she is beautiful.*

Soon afterward, a cyclone hit the coastline north of Port Hedland. The news was lackadaisical about it: the reports described the affected area as uninhabited—somehow overlooking the 500-strong Aboriginal community of Strelley Station. The day after the cyclone, Adele was contacted at work by Civil Defence who reported that, on a flyover of the community, they saw a cross laid out on the ground signifying a need for medical assistance. Adele and the doctor were despatched to the area to render what assistance they could. A Civil Defence vehicle accompanied them so that, if either became bogged, the other could drag them out. It was a terrifying drive: the very first creek they crossed, the water rose to the door handle and the current was very swift. Once off the main road, they were forced to crawl through the devastated landscape in low ratio. It took forever to get where they were going.

They eventually reached the Strelley Station clinic, miraculously unscathed among the ruins of the houses, and found the women gathered outside it, wailing. Lying inside on the bed was the lifeless body of baby Mary. Her mother, sitting beside her, reached out to Adele and tearfully told her that they were all sheltering in a strong communal building and that she'd had little Mary in her arms when she just stopped breathing.

The mother's note had been right: baby Mary was beautiful.

It was the final straw. For her sanity, Adele decided she and Shannon would return to New Zealand. Her thought at that stage was that she would train as a midwife and return to Australia. At her farewell, her colleagues told her they'd been taking bets on how long she would last back in a hospital setting. It is true that her reintegration was tricky at times: she had become sensitised to racism and to the subtle ways in which institutions and policies entrenched it. Nor after seven years in the frontline of community nursing was she shy about expressing her opinions on injustices wherever she found them. But what kept her going and ensured she proved her former colleagues wrong was her passion for midwifery. As a community nurse, she had felt helpless in her work with women, unable to change the way society treated them. Midwifery offered her the chance to advocate for choice and control in some of the most important moments in women's lives. She developed a belief that the key to health lay at the foundation of life and that the key holders were mothers.

Adele's own mother was unsurprised that she had found her vocation in midwifery, but she thought it had less to do with philosophy than with genes. When Adele's great-great-grandmother, Eliza Carrington, was widowed in 1890, her husband, Wellington, left her destitute with five children. To support her family, she returned to her profession as a Taranaki midwife. From the age of about thirteen, Eliza's daughter—Adele's great-grandmother—assisted Eliza at births and became a lay midwife. She then assisted at her own daughter's—Adele's grandmother's—births. Adele's mum occasionally joked that if Adele, as a child, had asked her the age-old question 'where do babies come from?' she would have replied that her gran brought them in her bag! Every time her grandmother came to visit, a baby came soon afterward. When she is sitting quietly with a mother in childbirth, Adele often thinks about this long line of her forebears who have performed the same ancient service, and of the thread that connects women and midwives through time.

After completing her training, Adele consolidated her midwifery practice working for two years at St Helen's Maternity Hospital in Auckland. Although the midwives at St Helen's had a considerable amount of autonomy, many aspects of practice were still controlled by the bureaucracy, and Adele's spirit chafed against it. In the end, her heart remained in the community, and when she saw an advertisement for a combined Public Health and District Nurse and Midwifery position on Great Barrier Island, her fate was sealed.

One of Adele's first experiences working with Ivan, the doctor, is the happy occasion of a birth. She has been on the island for less than a month when Ivan contacts her and asks if she will support him as midwife when he attends the birth at home of a local's baby. Neither Ivan nor Adele have attended a home birth, and this is a home birth with a difference: it is going to happen on Aotea, a remote island a long way from secondary support.

'She did not really give me much choice,' Ivan tells Adele. 'She said, "Well, doctor. I am pregnant with my third child. The first two were born at home, so I would like to know if you will come to the birth. If you don't, it will just be me and my husband because I have got no intention of going to the mainland."'

'Well, I'd be happy to come along, if I can get permission,' Adele says.

She phones the Director of Public Health Nursing in Auckland. They talk through the possible issues.

'I am experienced,' Adele says. 'And, of course, being a midwife is part of my job description out here.'

'OK,' concedes her supervisor. 'But we were thinking more that you'd be attending unexpected births rather than planned births.'

They talk some more. Adele likes this particular supervisor. She has been to the Barrier and, more than most, she understands what Adele's position involves. She also has more respect than many of the others in head office seem to for Adele's professional skills and judgement. 'If you and Dr Howie think that it's within your scope, then I'm happy to give permission.'

Adele lets Ivan know, and Ivan lets the mother know. Panic sets in! Both Ivan and Adele are products of the 1980s hospital system, which takes what in technical language you would call a 'biomedical risk-averse' approach to childbirth, rather than regards it as a natural process and presumes, in the absence of indications to the contrary, that it will go smoothly. It is hard, even for someone with Adele's firm convictions—she believes that if ever there is a moment in a woman's life when she should have the right to control her situation it is childbirth—to shake the precautionary mindset.

The woman lives in an isolated bay with no road access, power or telephone, so Ivan and Adele persuade her to find somewhere closer, so that if an emergency arises they will have some chance of summoning assistance in time. A friend offers her house. That is some comfort.

As the time draws near, Adele is in a state of constant, low-level anxiety. She phones a colleague on the mainland who has made home births something of a speciality, and asks what the procedures are.

The other woman laughs. 'There are no procedures. Every home birth is different. You just go with what the mother feels she needs to do. Really, it's her tea party and you're just there to pour the tea.'

This is cold comfort to Adele, who has only ever attended hospital births, where the entire process is homogenised. She arranges to travel over to the mainland and observe one of her colleague's births, but each time the opportunity arises it is impossible due to Adele's other commitments. Before she has a chance to gain any prior experience of home-birthing, the day is upon them.

Adele gets the call. Most of what she will need—instruments, linen, bowls, plastic for the floor, a baby resuscitation bag, gloves and absorbent pads—is in the 'birth pack' that she has already left with the mother, in case the birth happens before she can get there. She sets off. She can't prevent vivid scenes of obstetric emergencies flashing across her mind, and she has to will herself to be calm.

Her inner turmoil is in stark contrast to the scene she finds when she arrives at the house. Ivan is already there, talking softly with the supporters. The woman is sitting quietly on the floor in a warm room, in the lotus position and using yoga breathing to ride through the contractions.

It is not long before she looks at Adele and calmly announces, 'I'm ready to have the baby now.'

They go through to another room where Ivan has spread all the linen from the birth pack over a table in front of the fire. The woman sits down and, with her six-year-old daughter holding a mirror for her, she gives a few pushes and brings a baby boy into the world. Even the baby is calm and breathes immediately.

Ivan and Adele look at one another in awe, feeling a bit superfluous. The placenta follows routinely a short time later. The worst thing about the birth was that far more linen than was necessary was soiled in the process. Because the boat that took the laundry back to the mainland for washing and sterilisation only came once a fortnight, Adele had to give it a preliminary wash, a laborious process on Great Barrier. They quickly learned to make as little mess as possible.

She and Ivan cross tracks regularly. The rules segregating the public and private medical systems have created a paradox on the island. The nurses are paid a salary, whereas the doctor is reliant on government subsidies and patient fees. Therefore, if Adele immunises a child whose parents have had difficulty accessing the doctor, she is aware that this is effectively removing income from him and threatens the viability of his practice on the island. If Ivan resents this kind of toe-treading, he never shows it, or lets it undermine the team approach that Adele feels Ivan, she and Nancy are developing: it is simply a practical necessity that they are called upon to assist one another, and to share patient information in spite of the rules that discourage it. One day, in a meeting with her superiors in Auckland, Adele is questioned closely about how much contact she has with 'the doctor'.

'Not much.' She shrugs, although the truth is somewhat otherwise. She feels there is no point starting a debate over the rights and wrongs of interacting with Ivan when there is really no alternative. Adele refrains from asking how much practical support they are prepared to give her—would they, for example, supply their private numbers so that at two in the morning she can call them for advice about a patient? That is what Ivan is prepared to do.

Besides, by now, Ivan has brought a wife—another nurse and midwife—to the island, and with Leonie fast becoming a friend, another layer has been added to the relationship between Adele and the Howies.

Chapter 4

DISCOVERING PARADISE

A terrible noise wakes Leonie. It is her first week on the Barrier as Ivan's wife, and they are asleep in their small house at Kaitoke Beach—or at least, they were. The house is little more than an unlined, board-and-batten box with an upstairs loft bedroom, and it tends to amplify noise. This noise doesn't need any amplification. Both of them lie in the dark—which is absolute—trying to work out what is going on. There is metallic clattering, booming, banging, all interspersed with shouts and hoots of laughter.

'What the—' Ivan says. 'Is it Charlie's cows, do you think?'

There are no fences between the neighbouring properties and their own. But a particularly loud bang is greeted with an unmistakeable roar of what sounds like someone in pain. Ivan has decided a major emergency is happening. He is up and has grabbed his medical bag and is all ready to race outside, apart from the fact that he has not put his clothes on.

Leonie has realised what is happening. As she, too, scrambles to get dressed, hopping around with one leg in her jeans, she tries to explain.

'We're being tin-canned,' she says.

'We are what?' Ivan is nonplussed.

Leonie is having to reach far back into her memories of life up in rural Northland to recall what she knows.

'When someone brings a new bride home, everyone marches up the road banging saucepans and tin cans to serenade the couple to wake them up.'

She can sense Ivan staring at her in the dark.

'Why?' he asks at length.

'To wish them good health and to show support. Then it evolves into a party.'

'But we haven't got anything to give people.'

'I don't think that matters,' Leonie says, and she is right. They race to finish getting dressed and quickly swing open the door. There is a rousing cheer from the crowd assembled outside. Somehow they all pack into the house, all 23 square metres of it. Candles dimly light the scene —lots of big grins, people they know well and some Leonie has yet to meet—and there is no shortage of food or drink. Island hospitality is legendary and this is Leonie's first real taste.

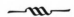

Over the years, people have often asked Leonie why she became a nurse and did not 'do medicine'. The answer is that nursing simply fits best with who she is. She flirted with the idea of becoming a doctor in her late teens, but the financial demands of medical school were probably always beyond her family, let alone her. But one of her most vivid memories as a child was sitting excitedly in the dark, watching an image flickering on the screen in her rural school as part of a series of sessions on the amazing things that people can do 'when they grow up'. This was the first to grab her attention.

The film followed a nurse sitting on the ground in an African village, white veil and all, teaching the children about handwashing. The nurse spoke also about caring for several unwell children in a small hospital in a nearby town. Something took root in Leonie's mind, and for weeks afterwards her thoughts kept returning to the nurse in that film.

That's it, she decided. *That is what I want to do.*

She felt she could just about reach out and touch the job, and in her naiveté she thrilled at the thought of the romance and adventure of a life like that—exotic places, doing good. For several years, she fervently knitted peggy squares and made stuffed animals for Junior Red Cross to send across the seas 'for the needy'. What she sees, looking back, is that the film and her imaginings about nursing fed into a deep-seated desire she harboured to care for people. The hallmark of a good nurse, her mother would tell her later, was to be 'caring'. Her dad just seemed delighted with the idea that she would want to be a registered nurse like her mum.

Through this phase of Leonie's life, her mum was providing for her the very model of the 'rural nurse', caring in an unpaid capacity for their extended family and unwell community members. If someone asked for help, there her mum would be. Her mum's willingness to always be available was never questioned by her family or neighbours. When she looks back, Leonie sees that she has always placed upon herself the same set of expectations in her practice that her mum placed upon herself. Such dedication can be an asset to a rural nurse—but it can also be a two-edged sword.

When she finished school, Leonie and her best buddy embarked on what they imagined would be a grand adventure out of their rural comfort zone and among all the excitement and glamour of Auckland. And, in fact, Leonie loved the years of hospital-based training and staffing. No sooner had they been awarded their nursing badges than they departed on the 'overseas experience' that New Zealanders regarded as compulsory. They bumped their way across Asia to eventually arrive in Europe via Afghanistan, Turkey and Iran. They settled in southern England, and registered with a nursing bureau. New Zealand nurses—then as now—found themselves much in demand, and, with work easy to come by, they divided their time for several years between stints nursing and discovery trips abroad.

Bureau work was stimulating and varied. One post she had was as nurse at a Butlin's Holiday Camp at the seaside resort town of Bognor Regis. Here, she was the night nurse in sole charge of a very well-equipped emergency clinic within the complex. On her first night, the management locked her in with strict instructions not to open the door to anyone other than a security guard. Under no circumstances was she to visit a room without a guard.

What have I got myself into? she wondered. This was supposed to be a fun place where people went on holiday, not a maximum-security compound.

By the time she had dealt with pairs of staff members on two occasions who had sustained injuries from bouts of fisticuffs, she began to get the drift. On each occasion, there were security guards hanging on to each protagonist for dear life. She needed no further persuasion to keep the door locked and bolted.

When eventually she returned to New Zealand, Leonie trained in midwifery, motivated by the same urge to care that had called her to nursing. Once she had consolidated her midwifery, she chose a job that served to give her a solid grounding in community health. She became increasingly conscious of Māori health needs and the way in which the health system was failing to address them. In 1984, she attended Te Hui Whakaoranga, a large, national hui where issues surrounding Māori health were aired. Here, Dr Mason Durie spoke on Te Whare Tapa Whā, his conceptualisation of the Māori belief system, and the way in which Māori approaches to health flowed from principles grounded in mātauranga Māori (simplistically defined as Māori ways of knowing) and te ao mārama (the Māori world view). Not only did she learn much about her patients; Leonie also began to understand better who she was, embracing at a deeper level her own Māori heritage and tikanga, guided by her older sister, who had trodden this path before her.

Her nursing and midwifery role saw her work as part of an urban health team that worked on holistic and Christian principles. The suburb in which they were working had, at that time, a wide range of health needs, and because she lived (and worshipped) amongst her patients, this was her first experience of the complex relationships that are such a big part of rural nursing. She revelled in it, and there is no doubt that it played a big part in shaping her for her role on Aotea, quite apart from the fact that it was in 1980, during this time in her life, that she first met and worked alongside Dr Ivan Howie.

Ivan always intended to be a doctor, but also wanted to study theology. After graduation from med school, he completed a degree in Divinity. He served for a time as a Baptist minister, but medicine called him back. He worked (among other posts) in the same Christian community health team as Leonie and—though she didn't know it at the time—would much later become her partner in life.

In the meantime, though, the dream of being the nurse in that flickering black-and-white film was still there, and it drew Leonie towards the idea of missionary nursing in a developing nation. When she was asked to be part of a community health team in Nepal, it seemed truly providential: she believed that, in this role, she would get the chance both to put into practice the cultural and spiritual understanding she had lately gleaned, and to learn. It would be a short-term taste of what might lead to a longer commitment. So she stuffed her belongings in her pack and set off for the Himalayan foothills to join the community health team based in Tansen.

—⁓—

When people ask Ivan how he and Leonie came to be married, he usually tells them that she had suffered a head injury and he struck while her judgement was impaired. The first part is true. In 1984, Leonie was recently back in New Zealand from her stint nursing in Nepal. She re-joined an all-woman crew racing a little 7.7-metre yacht in the Royal Akarana Yacht Club's Winter Series—lots of fun and good for the soul. At the time, although engaged again in the community nursing role that she loved, she still had thoughts of university, then returning to Nepal. One day out on the water, she neglected to observe one of the cardinal rules of yacht racing: duck when the boom is swinging. The subsequent concussion had a lingering effect.

While she was still in the process of rehabilitating from that trauma, as well as from a painful relationship break-up, she went with a group of friends in the summer of 1986 on a yachting trip to Aotea. They spent most of their time in the waters surrounding Port FitzRoy, and then those who had to return to Auckland all squashed into a taxi travelling down to the airfield at Claris, 60 minutes away. While she was waiting to board her flight, she spotted a familiar face. It was Ivan. They got talking and reminiscing about the three years they had worked together in Auckland. Leonie is amazed at how the years have flown by, especially when she hears that Alastair, Ivan's son, is now at high school. Leonie learned that Ivan had now been working as Great Barrier Island's sole general practitioner for six years. For the first three, he had commuted from Auckland—that much she knew as their paths had crossed through work. Then he had taken the plunge and settled permanently on the island near Kaitoke Beach, and he and Leonie had fallen out of touch. He told Leonie he was running his practice out of a caravan. It sounded adventurous and she was intrigued.

If you ask Leonie how she came to be married to Ivan, she will tell you that he was a GP working on a remote island who needed a nurse but could not afford to pay for one: marrying one was his only option. It is true that the relationship began somewhat tentatively from her side. But in March 1986, Ivan invited her back out to the island to spend some time with him, and she found herself accepting.

That trip—the first official 'dating' expedition—didn't start so well. Just as the little commuter plane she was on was about to take off, someone shouted from a seat at the back of the plane that the back baggage door was flapping open. The plane stopped with a lurch, and the cabin filled with the roar and whine of the engines and the smell of fuel as, right there in the middle of the Auckland International Airport runway, the pilot opened his door, leaped out, ran to the back and banged the offending door shut, then sprang back into his seat as though this were an everyday occurrence. They were in the air a few seconds later. Leonie prides herself on her sense of adventure, but at that moment she wondered what else might malfunction on the way over.

Ivan met her at the airfield at Claris, and she wasted no time in telling him about the 'drama'. If she was expecting him to be mortified and sympathetic about her apparent near-death experience, then she was wrong. He launched into a series of tales of the joys of commuting in small planes, and told her that it was all part of the experience of island life. Trying to be reassuring, he added that he regularly shared the cabin with cats and dogs, and had even flown with a goat and chickens.

'The airline is great,' he said enthusiastically.

If this was meant to be reassuring, it didn't have the desired effect. Leonie was already dreading the return flight, and was tempted to agree with those of her friends who thought she was mad contemplating a relationship with someone who lived in such a remote place.

But Leonie survived the return flight, and many subsequent flights. The relationship flourished.

If Ivan is being serious (he is well known for his fondness for a joke and a propensity to pun) and you ask him how he came to be with Leonie, he will tell you that he knew from the outset that she was the one. He suggested they should get married. Leonie found herself readily agreeing. She realised she had fallen in love with Ivan. She had grown up in Northland and, despite having lived in Auckland and overseas, she was a rural girl at heart. Aotea and its wonderful, ruggedly individual people called to that part of her. She and Ivan were married in November 1986, and soon after that Leonie set off to join him in paradise.

'Right. Welcome to the Tryphena Medical Clinic.' Ivan proudly opens the door to the old school building, an old kauri affair, two rooms—well, a room and a kind of porch or anteroom annexed to it—fitted out as a perfectly functional medical clinic by a committee of dedicated locals. It is relatively sparsely furnished and equipped, but it serves the purpose. Ivan holds regular clinics here, down in the southern part of the island, over the hill from where he and Leonie live on Kaitoke Beach.

Ivan turns the radio on. It echoes loudly in the empty wooden space. 'I do this,' he tells Leonie apologetically. 'It's the only way I can prevent my conversation being heard in both rooms.'

'What do you do for special equipment?' Leonie asks, looking around.

Ivan hoists his medical bag. 'I have become adept at carrying all I need.'

Soon the patients start to arrive. They know about Leonie, and they greet her with a mixture of curiosity and what she begins to realise is proprietorial satisfaction. She has married 'their' doctor, so she has chosen to be 'their' nurse. Her decision to marry and live on the island is a gesture of commitment to them—although she didn't realise this at the time.

Mostly Ivan works behind the closed door of the main room while the porch serves as the waiting room. In the first few months, Leonie is confused about what her role is, as she is used to working in a busy urban practice with her own space. But here, unless Ivan specifically needs her, Leonie realises she is best employed sitting on the porch and just getting to know the locals and listening to their incredibly interesting stories. She feels like a fish out of water, not understanding who is related to whom or why two people could be sitting in the waiting room talking to her but not knowing each other. She introduces them.

'Oh, I know his name. I've been hearing his name hereabouts,' one older local says of another, with whom Leonie is sitting. 'But we've never actually realised who the other is.'

'It's true,' the other confirms. 'Probably because he lives in the south and I am more in the centre of the island.'

'How long have you lived on the island?' Leonie asks.

'Ooh, it must be about twenty years,' replies the first.

'It would be,' says the other. 'I first heard your name about twenty years ago, but I've been busy working on my land.'

She learns that Tryphena was named after a Sydney-built sailing vessel that used to ply between this sandy bay at the island's southern end, Auckland and various other international ports, mostly trading kauri logged from the island's forests. She learns that the building she is in was built in 1884 and served as the local school until 1939, when a new school was opened. Salted throughout the conversation are the names of some of Aotea's oldest families: the Medlands, the Blackwells, the Sandersons, the Grays and others. There are families with those surnames still living on the island. Locals use names as though Leonie will have heard of them already.

She is called away from one fascinating story by Ivan, who asks her to suture a wound while he is attending to the deep gravel graze on another limb. She quickly finishes this task and looks around for the autoclave to sterilise her instruments, forgetting for a moment where she is. Then she spies the water bath steriliser 'of sorts' and remembers.

Leonie raises her eyebrows, but she recognises a practical yet sterile arrangement when she sees one. She and Ivan are eking out a living, their total income considerably less than Leonie was earning on the mainland.

On Wednesday, they drive in Ivan's iconic and durable light blue Holden HQ up north to the nurse's cottage in Port FitzRoy for the northern clinic. The car bumps and rattles its way over the saddle beside Hirakimata (Mount Hobson). At this time, in the mid-eighties, it takes the Howies just under an hour to reach Adele's clinic. Although it is a relatively small island (the Barrier covers 27,360 hectares, and is roughly 40 kilometres long and 10 kilometres wide at its widest point) with a population at that time of just over 850. Getting around is hard in the mountainous terrain. The drive along the winding metal road, through the native scrub and forest that covers 88 per cent of the island, seems to take forever. And Leonie has already seen enough to realise how little most of the population has in terms of income. Some are farmers or fishermen, and given everything costs more than on the mainland, and given the high costs of getting your produce to market, the returns are significantly less than on the mainland, and are often marginal. Leonie will often hear it said that farming or fishing out here is a way of life rather than a way to make a living. Most of the islanders are working hard to survive. Those fortunate to receive a steady income are aware of the privilege.

Adele is away doing Well Child home visits when they arrive at the nurse's cottage for the clinic, as she often is when the Howies make their regular visits. By contrast with the Tryphena Medical Clinic, Leonie finds the clinic attached to the nurse's cottage well equipped, and she notes with some envy that Adele has an entire room within which to work.

The Port FitzRoy clinic lasts most of the morning. Leonie really enjoys having the one-to-one time with the islanders. A good number of the FitzRoy people have come by boat from isolated valleys, bays and offshore islands. Leonie is bewildered with all the talk of these unfamiliar places. She resolves to get herself a good map and try to put places to the names at the earliest opportunity.

At the end of the morning session, they loop north of Port FitzRoy to reach Karaka Bay, just around the point from Rarohara Bay, where a large community named Orama Christian Fellowship is sited. A lunch is laid on—and then the Howies hold a clinic in the community's purpose-built sick bay. The community is a mixture of full-time residents and people who have come to Orama—which takes its name from the Greek word for 'vision'—to recharge their spiritual batteries. It is an ideal place for this, situated as it is behind a wide, tree-fringed lawn at the head of a beautiful, sheltered cove. But it is for the more secular comforts it provides that Leonie will come to love her visits to Orama. In the early years, the laundry facilities and the hot showers she can enjoy at the turn of a tap are bliss compared with what she has at home—a kettle boiled on the wood stove or a solar-powered shower (a bag laid outside to heat in the sun), or a cold shower, or a dip in the surf with a bar of saltwater soap.

When they are not at the southern and northern clinics, Leonie and Ivan are based at their 'practice facility', centrally located at Claris. Ivan was not joking when he indicated that the hub of Great Barrier Island's primary medical facility was a caravan. It is not even a new caravan but an older-style one, small and painted two-tone moss green. Ivan had pointed out that in its previous incarnation it had been the local fast-food outlet. He has set it up to suit his needs. He has a locked filing cabinet for all the clinical records and a hidden cupboard—also locked—for his supply of medications. Instruments are boiled over a gas burner in a stainless-steel lidded container for the requisite twenty minutes for sterilisation. There is a foldaway table that is almost never folded away, as it is usually littered with textbooks and assorted other papers. There are various cubby-holes and lockers, and each is filled with medical supplies.

Its other distinctive feature is the slight musty smell it perpetually has. There must be a leak somewhere—never bad enough for actual water to become obvious, but just bad enough to ensure there is always a damp smell. Ivan's attempts to locate and fix it have been to no avail. Over the years, Leonie's own occasional search will be fruitless, too.

The caravan is positioned directly beside the front door of their little house, so Leonie becomes accustomed—as Ivan already is—to their home being used as a waiting room or a sleep-over space for those needing to be cared for overnight.

From the huge window in their upstairs bedroom, they have a view of the airstrip way out over the sand dunes, so Leonie and Ivan can check the visibility during rough weather and at night. Sometimes they are called upon to report flying conditions for the mainland, and even provide a sketchy weather forecast. As Ivan explains to Leonie, if you can see the summit of a particular hill at the end of the beach, the cloud ceiling is high enough for a plane to get in.

Not that communications are any easier than they are for Adele at Port FitzRoy. Leonie and Ivan are on a party line, and one of the ten subscribers on their line is the public phone box at Medlands Beach.

'The operators always seem to know where I am,' Ivan explains. 'It's uncanny. I don't know how they do it.'

Leonie soon discovers the same. If there is an emergency, no matter where the Howies are, the phone will often go and the operator will ask the person who answers for Ivan or Leonie. And on the occasions when neither she nor Ivan is close to a phone, the operators simply hold messages until they get home or are in a position to receive them. Answering machines are just coming into vogue on the mainland; not long after arriving on the island, Leonie decides that the island system is far more efficient.

The downside, as Adele has found, is the lack of privacy for their patients. In order to maintain medical confidentiality on their party line, Leonie and Ivan often wait until eight o'clock, when the exchange is closed and the Claris public pay phone is switched over to the New Zealand international exchange.

One starlit night soon after Leonie took up residence on the island, an emergency arises that requires the patient to be urgently evacuated to hospital. Ivan treks up to the Claris phone box as usual, only to find that the operator has forgotten to switch the phone over. It simply rings in the empty exchange. Finding and waking the operator will take too long.

Fortunately, the local policeman lives close by. Ivan rouses him to see if he can help break into the exchange.

'Yes,' the policeman says without hesitation, and he jumps in the car and Ivan retraces his journey back to the exchange.

'Won't you need tools? A hammer or something?'

'Watch and learn, Ivan. Watch and learn.'

The policeman is in the process of showing Ivan how easy it is when they hear a car approaching.

'Oh no!' the cop hisses. 'Get down!'

They both drop and wait until the car has passed by. Both of them know it would take some explaining if the island GP was found breaking and entering under the expert tuition of the local policeman!

They 'effect entry', as the policeman would put it if he were writing the burglary report, the phone is switched over and Ivan is soon listening to the international operator saying, 'New Zealand here.'

The next day, they fess up. It would have been obvious for a detective anyway, as the doctor's and the policeman's sticky fingerprints are plain to see all over the glass. Fortunately, after that night, Ivan will never need to use his new-found burglary skills.

Just like Adele, Ivan and Leonie have a CB radio on at all hours of the day and night. The drawback is that the Taiwanese long-lining fleet, well over the horizon much of the time, are on the same frequency, and the radio will often squeal into life with no warning in the small hours of the morning with a staccato burst of rapid speech in a slightly off-key foreign language.

And of course, if they have no way of reaching them by telephone, the locals know where their doctor and nurse live, anyway. The method of contact of last resort is to bang loudly on the door.

Soon after her arrival on the island, Leonie wakes to just such a banging on the door. Her torch lights up two people, a young man leaning on an older one, who turns out to be his father.

'You'll be all right now, son,' the dad says. 'Doctor's got you. See you when you get back. I'm off!'

Before they can react, he has jumped in his truck and driven off into the night.

'Dad figured you would be shipping me off in the morning,' the lad says, noticing our confusion. 'He wanted to get back to sleep.'

'What happened to you?' Ivan asks.

'I crashed my motorbike,' he replies. 'My knee is really sore and I can't walk on it.'

They manoeuvre their patient into the caravan and, while Leonie holds the torch, Ivan cuts away the young man's jeans. The knee is badly swollen. Ivan examines it thoroughly, then applies a rigid splint and gives him something for the pain.

Leonie excuses herself and goes to make up a bed on the floor of their sitting room. Ivan helps the lad over and settles him on the bed, and just before she goes upstairs Leonie asks if he is going to be warm enough.

'I've got a jumper in my bag,' he replies. 'Would you mind grabbing it for me?'

She rummages in the backpack he was previously wearing and pulls out the jumper. Something falls on the floor, and she shines her torch on it. It is the biggest jumbo box of condoms she has ever seen! Leonie cannot help but glance at the patient, who is wearing a wry grin: he plainly had a far better evening planned than the cold one he is going to be spending on a makeshift bed on the Howies' floor.

Embarrassed for him, Leonie quickly stuffs the box back in the bag.

'Goodnight,' she says, and beats a hasty retreat.

'Night,' he replies, still grinning.

Soon Leonie becomes attuned to the sound of cars coming to the end of the road, which is inevitably followed by a pounding on the door. Late one night, she hears a vehicle arrive at a good clip, a reliable indicator of an emergency. There is a knock on the door. A man has brought his neighbour in. He is sitting in the vehicle with a blood-soaked towel clamped to his face.

Ivan leads him slowly into the caravan so he can examine the damage to his face. When the towel is removed, it is plain he has a horrific gash diagonally across his face, involving the bridge of his nose, his lips and cheeks but mercifully missing his eyes.

'He was up a tree using his chainsaw,' the neighbour explains. 'It kicked back on him. Then he amazingly got himself down and called for help. It was a bit of a drive to get him here.'

'You should have brought a photo of your favourite movie star!' Ivan tells the patient. 'Let's get started putting it all back together again.'

He numbs the affected area with local anaesthetic and then, with Leonie holding the gas lamp as steadily as she can, he begins laboriously stitching the shredded skin together, reconstructing the face. Leonie can only admire his handiwork, especially under the conditions: the patient is lying on one of the caravan seats. Ivan is half sitting, half squatting beside him and Leonie is leaning over his shoulder to provide the necessary illumination.

Leonie often has occasion to be pleased with her ability to detect late-night incoming cases, because it gives her a head start on waking herself up and getting dressed. Ivan is like a coiled spring and is out of bed the moment he hears a noise that is out of the ordinary. But it is a blessing that becomes a curse on the rare occasions that they travel off the island. Sleep becomes impossible in the city, as they wake every few hours whenever a loud car passes by.

The locals understand. They show their appreciation for Leonie and Ivan's dedication the way Barrier locals always do: they drop in with gifts of kai moana—crayfish, scallops and snapper—and even wild pork. Ivan and Leonie look after them; but more importantly they are looked after in their turn.

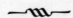

'He says he caught it in a winch,' George Mason relays by phone. 'He says he's lost one of his thumbs.'

'I need more detail please, George,' says Leonie. 'First ask him specifically where the amputation is.'

There is a short pause as George puts down the phone handset and picks up the radio hand-piece. Leonie can imagine many ears about the Hauraki Gulf listening to the drama unfolding on the public radio channel.

'The doctor's wife wants to know how far above your knuckle you've lost the thumb,' George says.

Leonie feels like rolling her eyes. George hasn't manned Great Barrier Marine Radio for all that long at this stage, taking over from his wife, Moira—but in all that time he hasn't stopped referring to Leonie as 'the doctor's wife'. It is a continual blow to her professional pride, but she has learned to live with it. George Mason has always been unfailingly polite, and he is a wonderful man: he has a long history of service to the island, being a farmer, a policeman and, most recently, a radio operator providing support to those boats in the waters surrounding Aotea and its constellation of outlying islands. But Leonie does sometimes wonder how much credibility she has as 'the doctor's wife' when she is relaying complicated medical advice through George. Do they assume she has any medical expertise of her own? Do they even follow her instructions?

'George says it's completely gone above the knuckle,' George relays. The fact that the commercial fisherman who has suffered the injury shares a first name with the radio operator has made the usually complicated three-way radio conversation even worse than usual.

'OK. Please ask him to cover the stump with a clean dressing and then elevate the hand as high as he can to stop it bleeding.'

'George, the doctor's wife wants you to keep your hand elevated and keep pressure on your thumb to stop the bleeding. Over.'

'And, George, ask him to bring us the amputated part of the thumb. Keep it cool somehow. Ideally, wrap it up in a clean dressing and place in a clean plastic bag and cool it with a slurry of ice.'

'George, the doctor's wife wants you to bring her the bit of the thumb that's come off. She wants you to wrap it in plastic and put it in the freezer. Over.'

There is a pause as Leonie raises her eyes to the ceiling, wondering how she can politely repeat the correct instructions to George without everything becoming a shambles. Freezing the thumb will be disastrous, as it will damage the tissues.

'No,' says George to Leonie. 'George says a goony bird swooped down and took the thumb.'

Leonie can imagine the delighted reaction to that piece of news broadcasted.

It is always a tricky balancing act between patient privacy and the need to know specific details when asking a patient to tell you exactly what is happening over the airwaves. And Leonie knows she is not just being paranoid when, for a week or two after this episode, boaties are sidling up to her and saying, 'So how did George get on? You know, George with the thumb . . .'

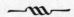

Many years later, Ivan and Leonie will eventually buy their 10 acres across in another valley, away from the beach—realising a deep-seated dream of Leonie's, who has remained a farm girl at heart, that her children can grow up as she did, surrounded by animals. The added privacy will be welcomed. When not on-call, they will be able to retreat from their busy lives on to the land and their new home. It will be a great change in their lifestyle.

Until then, Leonie feels they live in a fishbowl. Their home, of necessity, is always open to locals and visitors requiring their professional skills. Some days she feels, like Adele, that she is perpetually either working or being called out. There is no time for sailing or fishing—both too far from a phone. The idyllic Barrier lifestyle is right there, but hovering somewhere just beyond reach.

But, even during the frantic periods, Leonie knows that she has something special, and she will be confirmed in that knowledge as the years pass: she and Ivan share a unique partnership. Together they live and work all day, every day, the classic doctor–nurse story and yet as equals. They would not exchange this life together for anything.

Chapter 5

ARRIVALS

One thing that we have achieved on Aotea since Adele and Ivan attended their first home birth is the expectation that, in the absence of any indicators that the birth will be difficult or dangerous, it will happen on the island and probably at home. Not that we can take credit for this achievement: at all times, as in the birth process itself, it has been the mothers who have taken the lead. Some writers on the subject describe women who plan to give birth at home as ambassadors of good birth. The practice of home birth reminds the rest of us that birth at its best is natural, safe and healthy.

At first, the locals were appalled at the idea that we—the midwives, Ivan as the doctor, the mothers themselves and their support people— would be so reckless as to risk the lives of women and babies by allowing women to birth at home. But, with each successful, uneventful and joyous delivery, opinion has come full circle. The fact that up to half of the eight to ten women on Aotea whom we care for each year will give birth in their own island homes is now a source of considerable pride to the community. In fact, it is even beginning to flow on to the next generation of childbearing women, who are choosing to birth at home even if home is no longer on the island.

This is not to say that women feel under pressure to give birth at home. It is more a case that the community expresses itself willing to support a woman if she chooses to do so. And once the baby is born, it is enfolded by the community and owned, in a special sense, as 'our' baby.

Each labour is unique, and it is always extraordinary to watch as a new baby emerges into the world. No matter the struggles during the antenatal period or the birthing, we are left pondering, *How will this life unfold? What special things will this baby achieve as he or she grows to adulthood?* We have both been fortunate—Adele especially—to have watched over many island babies as midwives. These babies progress to become toddlers and preschoolers and, as rural nurses, we remain involved with their care. The watching and nursing continues through their childhood illnesses and their teenage crises to adulthood. Some, of course, are 30-year-olds now, with their own burgeoning families—so the cycle starts again.

The central person in a birth is the mother herself. This may seem so obvious as to be a truism, but sometimes it needs reiterating. The birth of a baby—in most cases, a natural event that a woman's body is capable of performing with minimal assistance—has sometimes become over-medicalised in modern society. This is not to deny that Western medicine has vastly reduced the dangers inherent in difficult births, but the fact that medical intervention can save lives has also given rise to the assumption that it can improve upon the natural process in every case. Over time, this assumption has been increasingly challenged.

Research has shown that a series of chemical events and processes occur in a woman's body when she gives birth. It is described as a hormonal cascade, and each step needs to happen at the right time and in the right way for an easy, natural birth to occur. It seems that one of the keys to triggering and maintaining this process is that a woman is in a familiar place and feels safe enough to birth her baby. The place that most women feel private and safe in is their own home, surrounded by people known to them.

Sometimes professionals are the only people present at the birth, assisting the woman and her partner. But most of the time numerous people come and go—mothers, sisters, close friends, children, aunts, grandparents. This could be overwhelming in a hospital birthing room, whereas in the home environment it is less so, as the woman can move to a private space in the house away from everyone. Close support people are vital, as they contribute to this sense of safety, and of course tend to continue their support postnatally with cooking, babysitting and housework. Usually by the time we leave the house, the whole community knows a baby has been born; often there is a sign put on the gate or at the general store. When British natural childbirth advocate Sheila Kitzinger describes the importance of 'god-sips'—support people who assembled to assist at childbirth in medieval times and who turned birth into an important social occasion (there are echoes in our sense of the word 'gossip')—she could have been describing the way it is done on Great Barrier Island.

The word 'midwife' comes from an old English term 'mid wyf', which merely meant 'with the woman'. Even as professional midwives, our job is to support the woman, who is the leader. After that first home delivery, Adele has assisted at many, many more. Each event has been individual, and she came away each time richer in knowledge and experience. She quickly learned that the best approach was to be open and flexible and to look at each woman and birth individually. She even learned to relax about the lists of risk factors that she drew up for each. Quite often, the women themselves have known instinctively what is right and safe for themselves. And they have invariably been willing to change their minds if Adele has shown herself prepared to compromise. Over time, her thinking has fallen into line with her convictions—that women have the right to choose, even where their choices could, from the outside, appear slightly risky.

As the lead provider of maternity services on the island, she has always had a team around her. In the old days, the team was Ivan. One day, he was sitting quietly in the kitchen while Adele attended the woman, and one of the children asked him why he was there.

'Well, Adele is here to help your mum if she needs it, and I am here to help Adele if she needs it.'

Quite unlike many doctors—especially in the 1980s—Ivan was happy merely to hold a torch to give Adele light. Once, the sister-in-law of the birthing woman asked Ivan to move out of the way so she could take pictures. Adele nearly laughed out loud, imagining how a hospital obstetrician would react to being pushed out of the way for photos!

While Ivan was more than qualified by postgraduate training and by temperament to perform the role of assistant, Adele was conscious that calling the sole general practitioner on the island away to a birth was often disruptive to the running of the medical clinic. She was grateful when Leonie stepped in to the role. Even so, in the early days, Adele often ended up attending on her own. Later, when best practice dictated that there should be two midwives for each birth, we began to work more closely together. Midwives have also come to the island to relieve when unforeseen circumstances have arisen, or specifically to be with women whom they have assisted at births elsewhere in New Zealand. From time to time, midwives have lived for short periods on the island and, where possible (if the women agreed), Adele has involved them in any births occurring while they were here. These days, Adele also has a rural nurse who supports her in her nursing practice in the north and is sometimes able to assist her with maternity care.

The island women and their families have allowed us to share an intimate part of their lives and this has strengthened us. We have met wonderful men and women present as support people who have radiated caring and love. We have learned new skills—massage, for example, from other women present at the births—and in turn have passed this knowledge on. We have witnessed the natural acceptance and excitement of children present at the arrival of a new sibling. We have been exposed to different music, languages, religious beliefs and philosophies of life, and we are the richer for it. We have shared food and cried and laughed with people we did not previously know well, and have built lasting friendships. We have learned that birth can occur in all sorts of places and positions, in differing amounts of light, with varying numbers of people present. We have witnessed how a community can rally around and give support to families, and how birth viewed as a positive and happy event can contribute to community well-being.

Community midwifery can be terrifying, exhausting, challenging and immensely satisfying. Mostly, when Adele asks women if they have any plans for the birth, they reply, 'No, I trust you.' In the old days, this made her anxious, because she did not feel experienced enough or worthy of this trust. Gradually, though, she came to understand that women being able to trust her (and leave her to feel the anxiety) freed them to give birth without fear, and that it was all part of a process that ended in a natural birth. No fear equalled no tension equalled a steady progression of labour, which equalled a woman easily able to cope with contractions and led ultimately to the birth of a healthy baby. Even so, after 31 years of community midwifery practice, Adele is still learning not to lie awake at night and worry—about decisions that have been made and about things that might happen—and simply trust the women themselves. All this time, and she is still learning.

Two births are imminent and Adele is experiencing her usual doubts, only at greater than usual intensity. One of them is a birth she has agreed to attend on an island off the coast of Great Barrier Island. Amber's* whānau is tangata whenua, and this will be her fourth baby. Her first birth, in hospital, was a set of premature twins who had a twin-to-twin transfusion—a condition where two foetuses share a single placenta and the blood flow is generally shared disproportionately. It usually has profound implications for the babies, and in Amber's case one baby died, and the survivor was left with cerebral palsy. Her second birth, that of her son, was on the mainland, and all went very well. This, her third pregnancy, has progressed smoothly, but Adele is thinking about the 30-minute boat trip to the island, and the weather, and about what happens if anything goes wrong. And what if the birth is at night, and she loses sleep? How will that affect her performance and judgement, if she is called upon to attend the other birth soon afterward? And of course, what happens if both go into labour at the same time?

The call, when it comes, is at six on a beautiful summer's morning.

* Not her real name.

Amber has been contracting since 4 am and is sending her brother-in-law to collect Adele.

At 7 am, she loads her emergency gear and extra pads, towels and linen into the brother-in-law's fishing boat. He throws the engine into gear and gives it a bit of throttle, and just as they are leaving the wharf, the glassy waters of the bay are disturbed by a pod of dolphins seeking out the pressure wave from the bow. No time to play, they roar out towards Man of War passage, between Kaikōura Island and the southern headland of Port FitzRoy. Twenty minutes after setting off, they hit the open sea. It is not calm (it rarely is) but the boat and skipper are well accustomed to these conditions and handle them effortlessly. As they reach the lee of the destination island, Adele sees two orca hunting the shallows for stingray, their distinctive, tall fins weaving above the shadows of their large bodies beneath the water. The skipper drops the engine to an idle and shifts out of gear and the boat glides into the wharf. The engine bellows as he gives it a quick squirt in reverse and brings them expertly alongside the wharf. He leaps off nimbly and drops a bight of rope around a bollard as Adele waits with her bag. She scrambles stiffly up on to the wharf. Twenty years ago, when she first visited Amber's grandfather on this very island, she jumped off just as easily as the skipper did. Now she can only envy him his agility.

Beyond the wharf, they pass through a barricade designed to stop wandering small children, and then walk up a steep path to the house. Adele was last here in her capacity as rural nurse just prior to the tangi for the family's grandad, and as she steps into the cool of the house she is surrounded by photographs. His photograph is there, with others who have gone before alongside the new generation coming forward. The morning is full of significance: life is ratcheting in its circle, and it is joining Amber to the spiral of the generations that have preceded her on this land.

It is twenty minutes to eight. Adele finds Amber coping with very long and strong contractions. Her waters are still intact. Her husband and mother-in-law are in attendance. As Adele is talking to Amber, another powerful contraction begins. She rolls on to her hands and knees, and her husband moves in and places a heat pack on the small of her back and lovingly rubs her back and shoulders. After a couple of minutes, it passes.

The interval between the contractions shortens, and fifteen minutes after Adele's arrival Amber moves from hands and knees to sitting. Adele is able to quickly take the opportunity to listen to the foetal heart through the smooth bulge of Amber's belly. There is no time to count, but the beat is reassuringly strong and steady. Twenty more minutes later, when she gets another chance to check immediately after a contraction—the time at which the foetus is under the most stress—she finds that all remains well with the baby.

Another contraction sets in. Adele sees that Amber is pushing this time, and she unhurriedly starts to pull on her gloves. She has only got as far as putting the left glove on when the head comes.

'Well, you told me your babies come at first push!' she says to Amber, and Amber nearly smiles.

Adele gets her other glove on and performs a quick examination. The umbilical cord seems to be around the neck, but loosely so. Adele leaves it alone, and with the very next contraction a well-toned baby boy emerges, who cries and coughs immediately. Adele unravels the cord, and passes the baby through Amber's legs and up to her. After a few minutes of skin-to-skin contact, Adele takes the baby boy and gives him a quick dry while Amber shuffles over to sit on the couch, whereupon Adele hands the baby back to his mother. Ten minutes later, Amber experiences another contraction. The cord has stopped pulsing. It is now safe for Dad to cut the cord, which he does, and then gathers the baby to him and takes his turn holding his son, skin-to-skin. Amber squats and pushes, and the whenua (the placenta) is eased out into a bowl. Adele examines it carefully for any evidence that it is only partial, or that there was a secondary attachment to the uterine wall. All seems in order.

She switches her attention to Amber, who has come through it well, too. Her perineum is intact with no need for suturing. It has been an unbelievably smooth birth.

'I'm so glad we didn't have to pack up the kids and get the boat and the car to get to Mum's place,' Amber says, as she sips a cup of Milo. Her mother lives on the mainland.

'True that,' her husband agrees. 'Ten hours, a real mission, and look at how easy it all was, right here.'

They look around appreciatively at their home, at the new layer of significance it has gained for their whānau.

Two hours later, all is normal with mother and baby—if the afterglow of a birth can ever be considered exactly normal—and Adele is back aboard the fishing boat. The reverse journey to Port FitzRoy is more sedate. The headlands with the swell crumbling at their feet and, beyond them, a few shreds of cloud around the summit of Hirakimata—it is a beautiful prospect. Adele thinks back to the beginning of this journey, blessed with dolphins and orca. It was such a perfect start to the day, a day on which a baby boy has started his own journey in the best possible way—an easy birth into a loving family at their home, with the photos of their ancestors looking on.

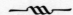

It is four years since Adele visited Jill's father in his isolated bay. Jill is now living in his bach—he has grown too unwell to live in such remote conditions and has shifted to the mainland—and she is in a relationship with the man who was clearing land for a house in nearby Allom Bay. The building of the house is underway, and they are expecting their first child (Jill's third). They contacted Adele because they are planning a home birth, possibly a water birth.

Now, late one autumn afternoon, Jill has rung to say the labour has started. Adele has had an early meal so that she can get to the house before dark. Shortly after she gets there, finding Jill glowing with excitement, Jill's partner also arrives home, just on dark. As soon as he has had his dinner, he and Adele begin the laborious process of heating water for the birth pool.

The birth pool has been hired from Auckland and shipped over on the cargo boat. Jill's partner has set it up in the kitchen of one of their two small baches and has the wood ranges in both baches going strong. Each range heats a small hot-water cylinder from a wetback, and to move things along he also has an open fire blazing between the baches with two big cauldrons of water heating there as well.

Just at the right time, the pool is full of lovely warm water. Jill lowers herself into it with a grateful sigh.

Ivan arrives. Adele called him as her backup, and the two of them retreat to another room where Adele tries to get some sleep and Ivan sits reading. Jill enjoys the bath until the later stages of her labour, when the sensation of water on her skin becomes uncomfortable. She climbs out, and it's soon clear the baby is on its way. The delivery is quite straightforward: a few pushes and a lovely, 7.5-pound baby is born at sunrise—a magical time of day, especially in such a magical place.

A phone call comes to say that Jill's father passed away that same morning: one soul passes out of their lives as another passes in.

It is two years on and Jill and her partner are expecting their second child. Leonie and Ivan arrive ahead of Adele; she asked them to attend when she learned Jill's waters had broken and labour had begun. They live closer to Okupu than Adele does.

This time, the trip to reach Jill involves a small boat across to Allom Bay. It is late afternoon but, unusually for the day of a birth, the weather is benign. Adele arrives to find the house finished. Jill's stonemason partner has crafted it with love and skill and it is truly a work of art.

We catch up quickly, and Adele learns that when the waters broke there was thick meconium in the liquor, likely indicating the baby has been or is stressed. Night is falling fast. We know that calling the helicopter to land in the dark would be challenging and Jill, her partner and Ivan are in full agreement not to take any risks. We call the helicopter, and farewell Jill and her partner.

They are back the very next day, with a healthy baby boy who was born within an hour of their arrival at the hospital, and Jill introduces this latest addition to her daughter and elder son.

We find that there is a slightly manic period between receiving the call from expectant parents and arrival at the house. This seems to produce a heightened awareness when we walk into the birthing room. You find yourself noticing things that you might not otherwise have noticed—the photos on the walls, the time of day or night, the other people present, the view outside, the lighting or, quite commonly, the music.

Adele in Western Australia, where she and Shannon moved two years after she had completed her nursing training. They lived there for seven years.

———

Adele (far right) quilting with friends. Adele learned to quilt when she arrived on Aotea, and these quilting sessions became a great source of emotional sustenance.

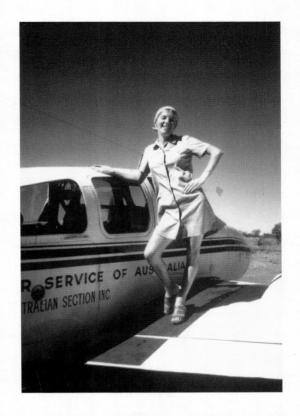

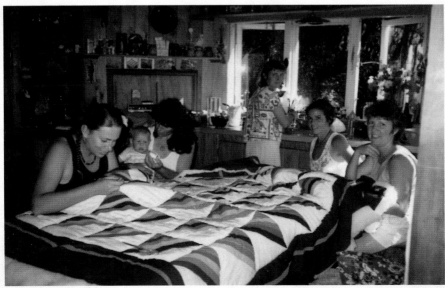

RIGHT

The Great Barrier
Island Howies in 1991.
From left to right:
Alastair, Amiria, Ivan,
Leonie and Jordan.

———

BELOW

The Howies' first home
and 'practice facility'
(the caravan) in 1986.

———

OPPOSITE TOP

The health centre
at Claris.

———

OPPOSITE BOTTOM

The nurse's cottage at
Port FitzRoy.

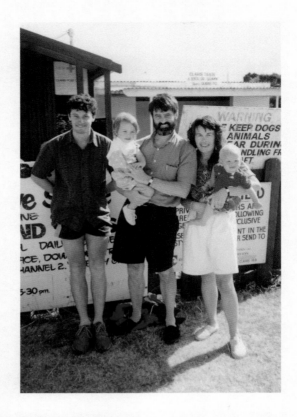

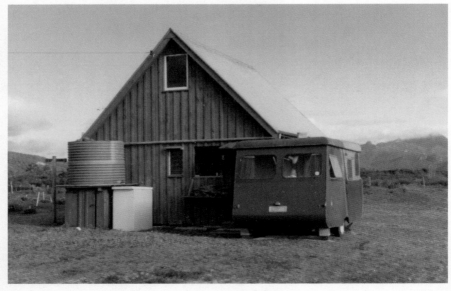

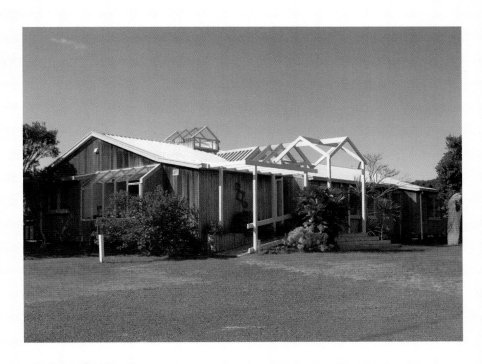

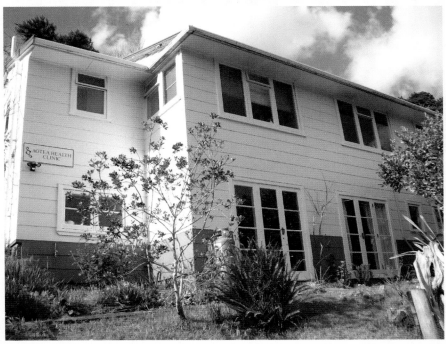

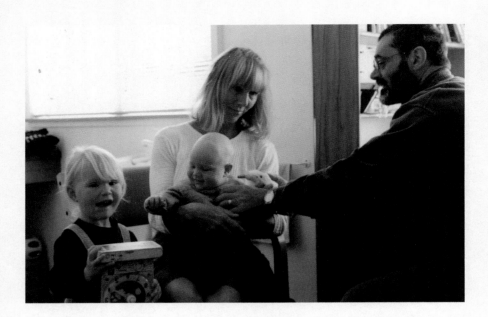

ABOVE

Jill visiting Ivan with her younger children in 1997.

———

RIGHT

Peter and Feral Cheryl ... before she grew into a gigantic sow.

———

OPPOSITE TOP

Some of the locals preparing a hāngī on Aotea.

———

OPPOSITE BOTTOM

Shannon and his business partner, Bruno, on the mussel barge in 1997.

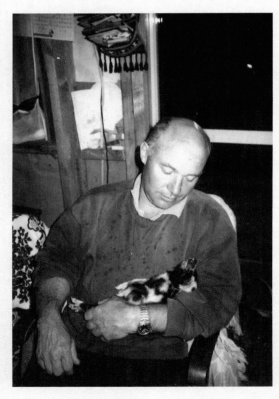

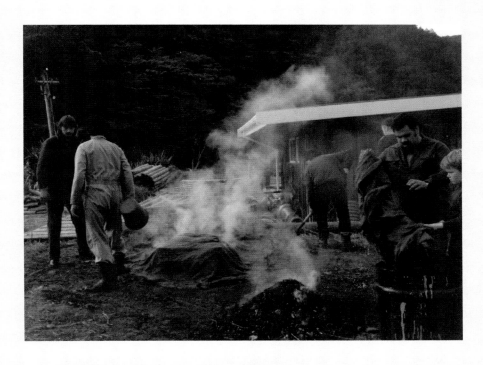

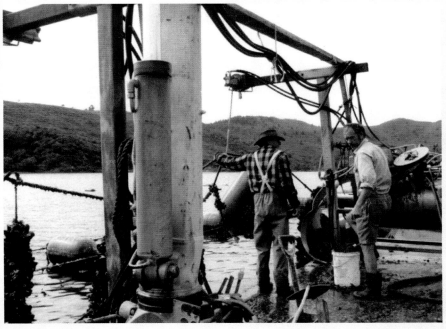

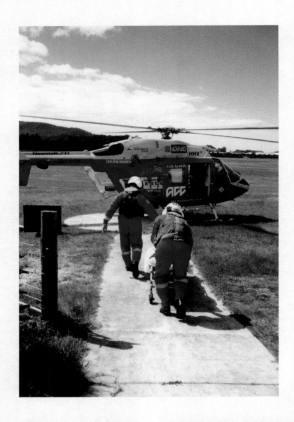

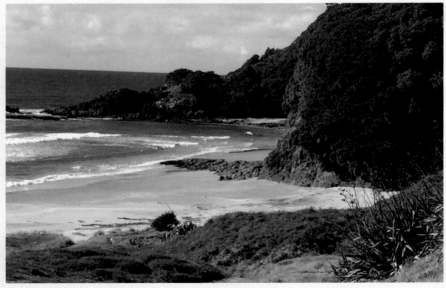

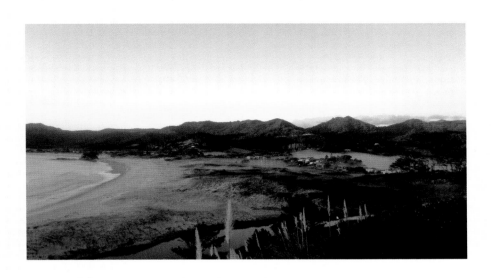

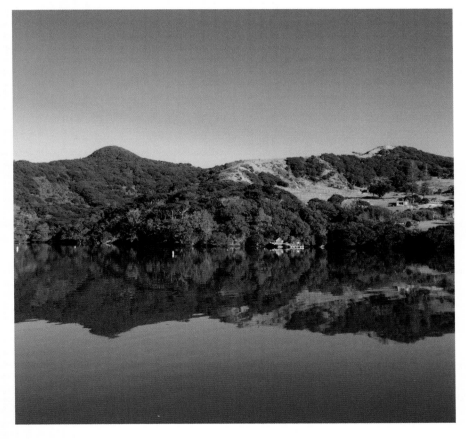

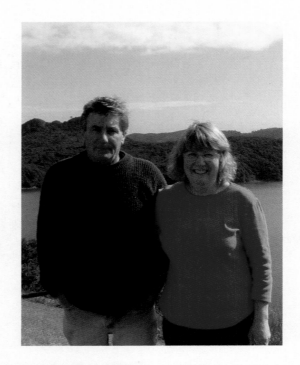

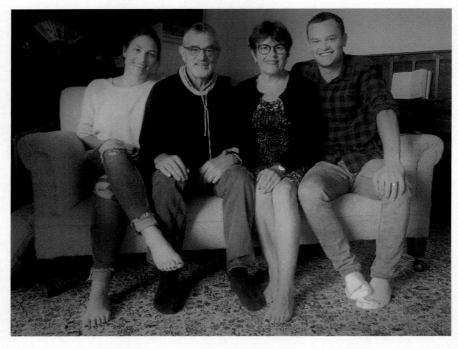

'Hi, Adele. It's Johann.'

Adele has been expecting the call. She checks her watch. It is 5 am.

Johann tells her that he and his wife, Kristie, have been awake since 2 am, when the first mild contractions set in. She was able to doze between them at first, but Johann has been flat out. Kristie wants a water birth, which is a tall order at the best of times on the Barrier. At Orama, where they are staying, their water heating is via a chip heater. Producing the necessary quantities of hot water to fill a birth pool is a challenge. They have a tiny hot-water cylinder, which Johann has drained, and even with the contents of the neighbour's cylinder he has still had to fill every available pot and pan and set them heating on the stovetop.

Kristie first presented to Adele at 27 weeks. She and Johann were missionaries in Africa, but had come home to New Zealand for the birth of their third child because they had been offered free accommodation and support at Orama in return for Johann working in the community. Adele had read Kristie's birth plan and its extensive list of requests with a sinking heart. She felt she was bound to disappoint Kristie, not least because she already had a week's holiday booked and paid for, her departure date just two weeks before Kristie was due.

But things had fallen into place. Kristie had been donated a birth pool from a business over on the mainland, and as the time drew near she and Johann had inflated it and leaned it up against the wall in a bedroom. Adele had called a relief midwife over from the mainland to cover for her while she was away, and Orama had donated accommodation for her. As it turned out, when Adele arrived back from her holiday she found Kristie still pregnant and the relief midwife relaxed and happy after a holiday of her own. Now, when Johann makes the call, Kristie is four days overdue.

After feeling initial misgivings at the very detailed birth plan,

Adele had adapted; by now, she knew that planning for the birth was the way in which many mothers seek to control the process. That sense of control can be essential to preparing the mother for a smooth delivery.

As she walks out of her door, Adele instinctively checks the weather. It is a crisp September morning, but it looks settled, which is reassuring. If there is an emergency, the helicopter will be able to fly.

As she makes the ten-minute drive up and over the hill to Orama, she visualises the birth and—because this is what she does—the things that could potentially go wrong. But when she arrives just before dawn and is welcomed into their home, all is serene. The room is warm with the toasty smell of a gas heater, and there is music. It is the music that Adele notices in her customary, hyper-aware birthing state: it is worship music—modern songs of praise, gentle and uplifting.

'I stopped worrying about being overdue,' Kristie is telling Adele, as the music swells in the background. 'I spent a lot of time by myself up on the hill looking over the sea. I just felt I needed space, you know? And I kept saying to myself that it was God's timing. I just sort of took the phone off the hook.'

Adele nods.

'I need the music going,' Kristie says. 'I get pretty vocal, and I don't want to scare the boys.'

Her two small sons are asleep in another part of the little house. Kristie is handling the contractions well, breathing calmly and shifting position now and again. There is not much for Adele to do but have a cup of tea and wait, listening to the music.

At about 7 am, Kristie climbs into the pool, stretches out and relaxes against the soft sides, a blissful look on her face. Johann climbs in as well, and presses on her back during the contractions.

One by one, the boys stumble, blinking, into the room. Once they have woken enough to absorb the news, Adele gathers them up with their little pre-packed backpacks and takes them to a neighbour.

When she comes back, Kristie asks her to check what stage she is at, and Adele finds her six to seven centimetres dilated. The contractions are strong and regular by now, and, between them, Kristie sings and prays aloud.

'I'm ready to push,' she gasps to Adele. Adele is surprised, but encourages her, and with the very first push the baby crowns. Adele knows Kristie wants to feel as much in control as she can, so she suggests Kristie touches the soft, downy head of her son. She cries out in delight, the sound as much a hymn of joy as anything on the stereo. With the next push, the baby is born into the warm, enfolding water. The vernix with which he is coated makes it hard for Kristie to get a hold of him, but Adele and Johann help lift him on to her chest. He cries, and they cover him with a warm towel. Mum gives him his first kiss—and the second, and the third—as Johann strokes her hair and gazes at his baby son.

Adele stands and watches. She is moved by this very spiritual birth to a couple with love and commitment to each other, to humanity, and to their Lord.

Later, Kristie and Johann had a fourth baby. This time, it was born in Benin in West Africa, and the only attendants besides Johann were the vultures watching from the doorway of their mud hut. The nurse who was supposed to assist had broken an ankle and couldn't attend. Nor could a New Zealand midwife who had raised funds to be there: she was still on the plane when the baby was born. Kristie managed the birth herself, and subsequently wrote about her African and Aotean birth experiences in a book called *Mud Hut Mom: My gentle birthing journey.*

Every now and again, Adele thinks about what 'home birth' really means—especially about what makes a home. She has attended births in all manner of places—a bus, sheds, in tiny houses, in houses still under construction, and in houses so remote from road access that they might as well have been boats at sea.

Now she is about to do the real thing.

She drives the same route she drove when she attended the vehicle over the bank. It is wet and wild again, which means there is no prospect of getting helicopter assistance, should all go badly, but she is just relieved to be answering this call as the baby is well overdue. She gets out and opens the huge gate in the predator-proof fence across the base of Kōtuku Peninsula. She drives through and climbs back out to close the gate again. The wind dashes sleety rain on the windscreen as she carefully negotiates the steep track: it has been vastly improved since that motor vehicle accident, for which Adele is very grateful. It is late afternoon by the time she is walking down the path to the narrow wooden jetty. She can hear water churning in the culvert beside the track. She is in full wet-weather gear: raincoat, over-trousers and gumboots, but she's shivering as she walks out on to the jetty.

It is a small sloop that Adele knows well from a previous birth. For Jacinda, the mother-to-be, and her husband, it is home. They had presented to Adele early in their second pregnancy and had told her about their dissatisfaction with the birth of their first child on the mainland. Jacinda had said she felt that she was subjected to unnecessary tests and procedures. She was not listened to, Jacinda explained: even the midwife seemed indifferent to what she felt was needed. Jacinda and her husband wanted a different experience, so they had sounded out Adele to see if she would be willing to attend the birth of their second child at home on the sloop. Adele had agreed. Now they were expecting baby number three.

Jacinda had a scan which indicated a definite due date. Armed with that information, Adele booked a holiday and set her departure date for three weeks after Jacinda's due date. That, she thought, would ensure the baby was safely delivered two, perhaps even three weeks before she went away.

Murphy's Law seems to apply especially to childbirth. The due date came and went. Another week passed, then another. Adele had begun to worry. The hospital was keen for Jacinda to be sent over, because induction is recommended if the pregnancy extends beyond ten days after the due date. The risk of complications, whether due to the size of the baby or the state of the placenta, soars. But Jacinda was perfectly confident that all was well with the baby and would be well with her, so Adele agreed that the plan to have the baby on the sloop could go ahead. And as it has turned out, the weather made it all academic. First, fog made it impossible for planes to fly. Then a storm front was predicted to cross the North Island. By the time the fog lifted, the front had arrived and Aotea was cut off in this maelstrom of wind and wintry rain.

Adele climbs over the lifelines and into the cockpit, the boat fretting at its mooring lines and the halyard slapping at the mast. The usual view out into the bay has been erased by the rain. Adele is relieved that things are finally in train. She is confident that Jacinda will handle the birth—we screen women carefully before agreeing to home births, and there are few risk factors in Jacinda's history—but the cramped confines of the boat promise to take Adele outside of her comfort zone.

She peels off her wet-weather gear under the cover of the spray dodger, and then ducks through the companionway into the cabin, where it is as though she has entered a different world.

Her own home was cold, but here all is warmth—there is a little wood stove throwing out heat—soft music and subdued light, and lavender scents the air. Jacinda's husband helps to set out Adele's equipment, and as she examines Jacinda she finds everything within easy reach. The contractions are weak and still quite erratic, so the birth is not imminent. Adele is able to go back home for a meal and some sleep before being woken by the phone.

'It's time to come back,' he says.

Jacinda's husband has made a beautiful wooden birthing stool from a diagram on the internet. Adele is not sure if this will work for Jacinda, but when the time comes she is prepared to give it a go, and it proves to be perfect for the birth. The baby comes through the birth canal quickly and cries loudly immediately after emerging. No problems at all—it is such a relief.

Adele gives the baby to Jacinda so that she can enjoy some skin-to-skin time. She has not checked to see if it is a boy or a girl, as the birth plan stipulated that Jacinda did not want to be influenced by the baby's gender as she enjoyed these first few precious minutes spent bonding.

Twenty minutes pass.

'Sorry, Jacinda,' says Adele, who feels she has been very patient. 'I just have to know. Do we have a boy or a girl?'

'It's a girl!'

It is a profound relief for Adele to have welcomed this little soul into the world, and the occasion seems to have special significance because, in the preceding days, there has been a death in community. Adele is set to attend the tangi in just a few hours. It is that circle of life again, the way things pass and are renewed.

'It's OK,' Leonie tells Jen, who has just apologised for failing to make conversational sense. Her waters broke a few minutes previously and without the cushioning forewaters present, the baby's head is now firmly in contact with her cervix. Where previously she had been chatting between contractions and taking deep, controlled breaths through them, they are now powerful and regular. No wonder she can't hold up her end of the conversation anymore.

Jen and her family are closely attuned to the rhythms of life on Aotea. Leonie has come to admire their down-to-earth practicality since she first met them.

Jen has been telling Leonie that, when the labour started, she decided she had best get a few things done before it got too far advanced, because she knew from her previous experiences that she would not have time for domestic chores after the delivery. So, contracting every eight minutes and with wide girth and all, she filled her bucket and waddled off down the path to water the row of brassicas she had planted just a few days previously. It has been a dry summer; she has painstakingly watered her prolific garden every day as her pregnancy advances. By now, she knows the whole routine of childbearing well enough to be able to judge what is in her power and what is not.

'It's OK,' Leonie reassures her again. 'We all understand you're a bit busy to talk.'

Soon a powerful urge to push overtakes Jen, and she scrambles to her mattress and on to her hands and knees. This is her third birth, and she knows from past experience that this is the best position for her. Another contraction overtakes her, and she groans.

'Why are you making that noise, Jen?' her three-year-old pipes up from the other side of the room. He has been standing in his cot, taking everything in.

'Because it makes me feel better,' Jen replies.

With the next contraction, she bears down hard and it is plain the baby is on its way. The older child, summoned by his dad, comes into the room. Everyone watches as, with a few hefty pushes, Jen births her new son, a brother for the children who are both watching, awestruck.

When the time is right, her six-year-old solemnly helps his dad cut the umbilical cord, separating the new arrival from his whenua. A few minutes later, the placenta itself is delivered, and Jen lies cradling her newborn son in her arms.

'Thanks for having the baby, Jen,' the three-year-old pipes up again. The excitement is over. He yawns cavernously, snuggles down again into his cot blankets and falls fast asleep. Everyone smiles. It is a special family moment that none of them will ever forget.

Certainly her eldest son does not forget it. Leonie learns later that the next day at school, he regaled his teacher and his classmates with a 'morning talk', using an impressive array of technical terms with insight and understanding.

You might call these typical Great Barrier birth stories, but in the end there is no such thing. And, of course, not everything runs so smoothly.

Adele answers the phone. She has been expecting to hear from Phaedra—expecting her voice tight with excitement and a little trepidation at what is about to start. But, from the moment Phaedra starts talking, something in her voice tells Adele that all is not well.

'There's blood,' Phaedra says. 'Lots of it.'

Phaedra had everything ready. She had the birth pool blown up and leaning against the wall of her bedroom. And she had been feeling restless. She got up at three in the morning and made a cup of tea. After sitting in the dark and sipping it for a while, she had told herself that nothing was happening, so she went back to bed and tried to go to sleep again. But she remained fidgety, and when she rolled over to try to get comfortable she was seized by a massive uterine contraction. There had been absolutely no warning signs— no niggles, no backache, no show (the passing of a 'plug' of bloody mucus that often precedes the onset of labour). Nothing. She felt a rush of liquid. Once the contraction had resolved, she stood to go to the toilet and felt the liquid curling down her legs. Deciding that her waters must have broken, she made her way to the toilet, holding firmly on to her girth. The liquid was flooding out, and when she had dabbed at it with toilet paper she saw at once that it was blood. Frank blood—bright red—had drenched the paper. Even as she stared at the wad of bloody paper in her hand, there was another gush spattering into the toilet.

Shit, Phaedra thought. *I should not be bleeding.*

Adele listens carefully to all of this. She tells Phaedra calmly that she will call Leonie straight away, as she is only eight minutes' drive away.

'Leonie will be there shortly, and I'm on my way, too.'

In the brief conversation that we then have, we are both aware that copious blood at this point in the pregnancy probably means an antepartum haemorrhage—a bleed before the baby is delivered, probably due to placental abruption, the early partial or complete detachment of the placenta. This is a full-scale obstetric emergency. Because the placenta supplies the baby with oxygen while it is in the womb, the prognosis for the baby is poor if it has detached too soon.

And with the baby unborn in a bleeding uterus, the mother's survival may be doubtful without emergency surgical intervention. Both of us know we do not have that kind of measure at our disposal.

Leonie wakes Ivan, as she may have need of his obstetric experience too. The adrenaline is ramping through her body. She is throwing on clothes as they discuss the situation.

'She had an ultrasound early, didn't she?' Ivan asks. 'Where was the placenta attached?'

'It was reassuringly high—well away from the cervix,' Leonie says. They both know that the high position in which the placenta was attached to the uterus is a good thing, because it rules out another serious cause of bleeding at this stage in pregnancy. Soon, Leonie and Ivan are running to their four-wheel-drive and are on their way.

They arrive to find Phaedra stripped of clothing and naked. A blood-soaked towel is jammed between her legs.

'There was another contraction,' she says. 'It was huge, and there was more blood.'

She is pale, alone, but holding it together. She was in the process of packing clothes for a probable trip to hospital when the latest contraction set in. Leonie is amazed. The practicality and good sense of the islanders has never ceased to astonish her.

'I felt the baby move,' Phaedra says. 'The baby's all right.'

Leonie and Ivan exchange glances. Leonie quickly ducks into the bathroom and sees more bloody towels, a pile of them on the floor, and blood splattered inside the toilet bowl. The blood loss is already maximal. There is a gasp from the bedroom as Phaedra undergoes another contraction. Leonie hurries back in. The contractions are coming thick and fast. Time is running out. They need to assess baby and mother and alert the emergency services.

Ivan checks Phaedra's vital signs while Leonie searches for the foetal heartbeat. So certain has she become that they may lose the baby that when she hears the beat—strong and clear—she is almost shocked.

'Phaedra,' Ivan is saying. 'Your recordings are OK. But can we put in an intravenous line to replace the blood you have lost?'

Leonie gently palpates Phaedra's pregnant abdomen. She can hardly make out the baby's head, which means that it is fully engaged in the pelvis. Sure enough, the vaginal examination finds her cervix fully dilated.

Ivan is already rummaging in his emergency kit when Leonie asks for his aid.

'Ivan,' Leonie says. 'The baby is on its way. Can you set up our resus equipment?'

Sure enough, a very short time later, with the bag of saline, the giving set and the IV needle still in their sterile packaging beside the bed, Phaedra rolls on to all fours and, with two massive pushes, the baby is birthed. Again, Leonie finds herself amazed to be seeing a pink, healthily breathing baby, rather than the limp, lifeless bundle she had imagined they might receive. She had been primed to begin resuscitation, but now she experiences a wash of pure relief as the baby wrinkles its face and cries lustily.

Phaedra lifts her baby girl on to her chest where the baby enthusiastically searches for her nipple. Phaedra looks as shocked at the speed of the labour and delivery as Leonie is at the happy outcome. Leonie forces herself back into action, and finds there is now practically no blood loss. Phaedra is shivering. Leonie drapes blankets over her and checks her blood pressure and pulse.

'Phaedra, your recordings are good,' she reports. 'I don't know if we need to replace your blood loss. What do you think?' she asks Ivan.

Ivan agrees to hold off. We wait.

Adele arrives, her face showing the fear she must have been feeling the whole way as she drove, the fear at what she was likely to find when she arrived. But this changes when Leonie tells her with a smile, 'Mother and baby are doing well and we're just waiting for the third stage now.'

Adele is offering her congratulations to Phaedra on her second successful birth when suddenly the lights go out. Everyone is sitting in total darkness. Ivan tells a joke. The genny is out of fuel.

We light up our trusty torches. Leonie's wrist is illuminated as she checks her watch. 'Fifty minutes since the birth,' she says. 'No placenta. But no more bleeding, either.'

Phaedra makes a small noise, and our torch beams swing to where the placenta is just now emerging. She gives a small push, and it plops into the basin, apparently intact, and with no further blood loss of note. So much for the 'abruption' theory. The birthing is now complete.

Adele remains while Leonie and Ivan drift off home to catch up on some sleep before starting their day's clinic in a few hours.

Phaedra recovers her energy quickly. She phones her family off-island to give them the good news.

Adele is happy with her recovery. 'Drink lots of fluid,' she says. 'And, above all, take it easy. You have lost a lot of blood and you may get tired easily. You will need the energy to care for your two girls.'

Phaedra nods.

But, soon after Adele has gone, Phaedra suddenly realises that the plane is due in a short couple of hours, and the place needs to be cleaned up. She sweeps the floor, spends time with her elder girl before she leaves for school, and deflates the birth pool.

'Fat lot of good you were,' she tells it ruefully.

Oh no! The genny!

Phaedra carefully straps her brand-new daughter into a car seat and straps the car seat into the car. The garage is just up the road. She is hoisting a jerry can out of the boot as the attendant approaches.

'Phaedra!' he says. 'You look like you're just about ready to drop!'

'Already have.' She smiles.

'No way,' he replies, but she points to the back window of the car. He leans to look. There is no arguing with what he sees.

'Oh my God!' he says, but what he really means is: 'Welcome, baby girl. Welcome to Aotea.'

Chapter 6

GROWING TOGETHER

As you would expect, our lives soon became intertwined. We were in the same profession and we had the same island as a workplace, but before long it ran deeper than that. These days, it runs deeper still, because we have shared experiences, and not just of the places and people we have in common. We have shared some of the triumphs and tragedies of one another's lives. We are colleagues and friends, and we are more than both of these things.

There are phrases bandied about in nursing and midwifery—boundaries, partnership, professional relationships. Things are supposed be tidy and clearly defined. But we have found that, on Aotea, boundaries shift like the tides, and all it takes is something unexpected to occur and we must react and readjust—a kind of rethinking on our feet. Nursing and midwifery are administered by separate professional bodies and have their own individual requirements of practice. In our situation they are not easily teased apart, and nor are professional relationships with one another and with our 'clients', and none of it can be entirely separated from friendships. But, in saying this, we have found that objective decision making cannot be distorted by our personal emotions. Once we place our figurative professional hats on, our other roles in someone's life become eclipsed for their sake—to keep them safe. Some episodes bring this home to you more than others.

Adele wakes in the early hours of the morning in the late eighties to the sound of quiet but insistent knocking on her door. She already has a fair idea who she will find when she opens it. Sure enough, after she has tugged on some clothes, she opens it to find Garth, the Okiwi telephone operator standing there.

'Sorry to wake you, Adele,' he says. 'Ivan just called. There's a woman in labour down in Tryphena.'

'I'll be on my way,' Adele says.

'Right,' Garth says, and returns to his car to drive back over the hill to Okiwi. As occasionally happens, Ivan could not raise the Port FitzRoy operator, so he turned to Okiwi. Garth was quite happy to make the eight-kilometre dash over the hill.

Adele is wide awake by now, the adrenaline pumping in her system. This is only her ninth home birth and, while there has been nothing to indicate problems, she is nervous.

It is 37 kilometres from Port FitzRoy to Tryphena, where Cathy lives. The road is rough, unsealed, very narrow, winding and—although it is a beautiful, clear night—very dark. At some points, there are steep drop-offs and there is no shoulder. But one good thing about driving on the island at night is that the wash of headlights alerts you to oncoming traffic. You do not have to crawl around the bends the way you do during the day. Adele is able to make good time, despite the awful surface.

All the same, she is an hour away, and her mind keeps tracking over and over the possible scenarios. A few days previously, she took the precaution of leaving a birth pack with Cathy in case the labour is fast: there is a chance she will arrive to find the baby has already been born. But there are other possibilities. What if she got the presentation wrong and the baby is breech—bottom first instead of head first? She runs through breech birth manoeuvres in her mind.

The schoolhouse and the airstrip at Okiwi pass by dimly. Somewhere, well off the main road, Garth is doubtless already tucked up in bed again.

What if the baby becomes distressed? Hospital assistance is at least 90 minutes away by helicopter. Adele goes through neonatal resuscitation procedures.

The farmland around Okiwi gives way to dense native bush, and Adele is half watching the trees on the bends for headlights, and half working on her contingency planning. What if there is a bleed after the baby is born? She rehearses in her mind the drugs and manoeuvres for post-partum haemorrhage.

The road enters the Awana Valley, another farming area. The black cattle here are escape artists, and Adele has to keep an eye out for them. At the southern end of the valley, she sees the cold blue gleam of surf along Awana Bay. Still no oncoming traffic.

Over the hill, the black expanse of the Pacific Ocean extends to the horizon as she leaves Aotea Road to wind along the roads named after the settler families. At Claris, briefly illuminated by the headlights, the small shopping centre and the main airport slide by along with the road to Ivan and Leonie's house. One of the roads is Walter Blackwell Road, and Adele is aware that Cathy is right now labouring in one of the old Blackwell family homesteads. Beyond Medlands Beach, the bush closes in beside the road again. Adele begins relaxation breathing and wills herself to keep her speed down on the corners. The bush eventually thins and then is replaced abruptly by housing, and she is passing through the outskirts of Tryphena. At the end of Medland Road, she indicates to turn left—unnecessarily, as there is nobody else on the road, and she has not seen another car since leaving Port FitzRoy. A short drive along Shoal Bay Road, another left into Blackwell Drive and she is there.

Dennis answers the door. He seems calm. He shows Adele through to the warm room in which Cathy is sitting on a mattress with Leonie, all smiles. Cathy is confident and prepared to welcome her new baby. Her contractions have been a bit erratic, and she asks if it is worth trying a mix of homeopathic remedies—caulophyllum, pulsatilla, hypericum and arnica. Adele has no objection to that, and they seem to do the trick. Before long, the contractions are strong and regular and everything is back on track again.

There are noises from somewhere else in the building. Adele is focused on Cathy and Dennis, but registers the sound. Someone, somewhere is in pain.

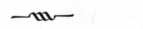

Earlier in the night, Leonie starts awake, aware that she has been woken by a noise, but unable at first to identify it. It is merged with a dream she has been having, so she is disorientated. She is drifting back to sleep when it comes again. It is a gentle tapping.

'Ivan.' She shakes Ivan.

He is awake in an instant, well used by now to waking at all hours of the night for some emergency or another.

'There is a weird noise,' Leonie begins, but the tapping comes again and Ivan is out of bed in a flash, grabbing a dressing-gown and thumping downstairs to the front door. Leonie listens.

'Sorry to bother you, Ivan,' a woman's voice says. 'It's Cathy. The baby's coming.'

Leonie is already out of bed and dressing when Ivan returns. He, too, starts throwing on clothes by the light of the 12-volt fluorescent tube running off a car battery. Leonie is wide awake by now. As she dresses, she clutches the bulge of her belly where her own baby—30 weeks along—is kicking ferociously, obviously none too pleased at the rude awakening.

Attending any birth is special, but there are new layers of meaning for Leonie in each of the births she has attended since discovering she was pregnant herself. Cathy is reaching the end of the journey of her pregnancy, and Leonie's awareness of the significance of the approaching moment is heightened by the fact that she is walking the same path. Cathy has asked Leonie to be her supporter. As she dresses, she feels again what she felt when Cathy first asked her: honoured, and a bit excited. It is funny, she has attended plenty of births before, both on the mainland and on Aotea, but she has always been there in her professional capacity as a midwife. But on Aotea she has observed at close quarters the role of supporter, and seen for herself how important it is to the labouring mother. Often it has been another woman who has walked the path before—a mother, a sister, a friend who has birthed before—and Leonie has been struck by the instinctual, almost spiritual connection between supporter and labouring woman, the way they seem to be able to communicate with one another without words, the way the supporter has seemed to be able to divine the needs of the mother-to-be without having to ask. You do not necessarily experience this when you are a professional, when your training is to remain detached and alert so that you can monitor mother and baby. Leonie hopes that she can turn off her midwife brain and be all that she needs to be for Cathy's sake.

She knows Cathy is prepared and focused, as have been all of the Aotea women whose births she has attended. Making the decision to have a baby on the Barrier is not done lightly, because when you do it you are aware that the nearest secondary-care facility is far enough away to be of little use in a real emergency. You are confident in your own body's ability to give birth safely. You are prepared to rely upon your own physical and emotional resources. 'Safe passage' is a term used in midwifery texts to describe how women prepare psychologically for pregnancy and birth—the mother's inward focus on the baby. This is apt, as it is a bit like putting to sea in a boat. On the island, we are further out to sea than most, quite literally. For this reason, it is only those who have developed the resilience to manage this emotional vulnerability who choose an Aotea birth.

The sound of Cathy's neighbour's car recedes into the night. Once dressed, Leonie fetches the 'birth-day' cake—a celebratory fruit cake—that she has baked and squirrelled away for the arrival of this baby. She pauses over the bottle of champagne she was planning to produce for the support team when it was all over. It is not good for breast-feeding mothers—or for pregnant women, for that matter.

Drat, she thinks, smoothing her hands over her belly.

They are dressed and about ready to go.

'We need to let Adele know,' Leonie says. 'Should we get Garth to drive over? He is such a light sleeper.'

'Probably the best idea,' Ivan agrees.

He loads his obstetric bag, his emergency bag and his medical bag into the Holden HQ as Leonie climbs in the passenger side, the vinyl of the bench seat smooth and cold against the backs of her legs. She feels the excitement tight in her belly.

They drive to Claris, where they stop at the public phone box outside the telephone exchange. Ivan gives the crank handle an expert twirl and, after a short pause, the international operator comes on in the almost imperceptible hiss of wire noise.

'New Zealand here.'

'It's the doctor on Great Barrier Island here,' Ivan explains. 'Will you put me through to Okiwi, please?'

'Certainly,' the operator says, and the quality of the silence on the line changes as Ivan is put on hold. Then the operator is back. 'Through now,' she says.

'Garth, it's Ivan. We need to get hold of Adele. Would you mind heading over the hill and waking her to tell her that the woman in Tryphena is having her baby?'

'Yes, sure. I can do that,' Garth replies sleepily. 'I'll leave right away.'

'Adele is alerted,' Ivan says as he climbs back in the car.

They leave Claris behind and wind over the hill towards Tryphena. Leonie has time to notice the sky—it is clear and ablaze with stars.

The shape of a car looms in the headlights, the bonnet up and steam seething out of the engine bay. Cathy's neighbour straightens up from where she is inspecting the engine. Leonie winds down her window as Ivan pulls up.

'Are you OK?' Leonie calls.

'Yes,' the neighbour replies cheerfully. 'Minor problem here. I'll be on my way soon.'

Ivan and Leonie press on, and just before four in the morning, they are pulling up outside Pōhutukawa Lodge, the old Blackwell homestead, which the Sages are running as a guesthouse. Dennis is at the door as they get out of the car.

'How is Cathy?' Ivan asks.

'Fine,' Dennis replies. 'We're all good.'

He shows them through to the sitting room, where there is a large mattress on the floor surrounded by all the necessaries—the birth pack, plastic floor protection, pillows, towels, a drink, newborn baby clothes and nappies.

'Hi, Cathy. I see you're all prepared,' Leonie says.

Cathy grins back. She looks happy and excited.

—⁕—

Dennis is on porridge duty when there is a loud knocking on the front door of the lodge.

Dennis opens it to find a worried-looking man standing there. There is the quite audible sound of moaning coming from a car across the road.

'Is Ivan there?' the man asks. 'That's his car, isn't it?'

'Yes, he's here,' Dennis replies. Ivan has already quietly slipped out from Cathy and come to see what is going on. The man looks tremendously relieved to see him.

'My wife's got stomach pains,' he says. 'Really awful ones. She keeps throwing up.'

Ivan accompanies him across the road, but soon they're back, both supporting the woman between them. She is in serious pain. Dennis has offered them a back room where Ivan can assess her.

Another car pulls up. It is Adele.

We compare notes with Cathy—everything is going well—and then Ivan calls Leonie out to help with his new patient. She passes from one dimly lit room to another and in the same instant goes from being maternity supporter to nurse.

'Rae has woken up with acute upper abdominal pain,' Ivan briefs her. 'It has been accompanied by vomiting.'

As if on cue, Rae leans over and is painfully sick into a bowl.

'I have discussed a plan with Rae to alleviate her pain and vomiting. Would you check these ampoules for the intravenous analgesia? How is our other patient?'

'She's good. Adele has everything under control.'

'Let's get a line in and try to get Rae stable.'

Leonie can tell Ivan is worried. He fires further instructions at her so fast she struggles to keep up. He then disappears quietly back into Cathy's room.

An hour later Rae is still writhing in pain, moaning and occasionally shrieking loudly. Despite the anti-emetic drug that Leonie has administered, she is still retching. Ivan frowns. The analgesia is also having little effect. Adjustments to the medication plan need to be made.

They are both conscious of the lack of communication with the outside world. They can't reach the Tryphena exchange. There is no VHF or CB radio handy. Dennis and Cathy's neighbour is clearly still tinkering with her car, because she has not returned.

Eventually there seems to be a bit of a let-up in Rae's symptoms. Leonie leaves and goes in to see how Cathy is faring. The contractions are close together, and everything is progressing well. After a few words of encouragement, Leonie puts her figurative nurse's hat on again.

So it goes for the next hour or so—Ivan and Leonie relaying each other in the two rooms. Towards six in the morning, as the dawn is brightening the windows, Rae appears to be more comfortable. Her vital signs are stabilising, and the drugs seem to have got the pain and nausea under control. Ivan feels she is stable enough to put her on the helicopter, just as soon as we can call it out from the mainland, to get her to Auckland Hospital for specialist surgical review.

Adele appears in the doorway. 'It's time,' she says.

We hurry back into the sitting room, where Cathy is very close to delivering her baby.

'Push,' Leonie urges her quietly, and so fully is she in the moment with Cathy that she finds herself bearing down in sympathy, her hands on her own rounded belly and drawing and holding her breath forcefully. She wills herself to breathe normally and to focus on Cathy. It would not do anyone any good if Leonie gave birth right next to Cathy!

The delivery is straightforward, and Leonie feels empathetic tears welling in her eyes as the baby emerges. Cathy and Dennis are dazed and glowing with the wonder of it. Cathy greets her baby and, after a few minutes, looks at Leonie.

'What were all the shenanigans next door?'

'You have a local as a guest who is unwell. Things have stabilised now, though,' Leonie reassures her. After all the drama of the emergency and the birth, all is quiet. Cathy asks for her parents to be woken—they have slept through it all—so that they can be introduced to their bonny 10-pound grandson, Jason. Sunlight—the first dawn of the baby's new life—is streaming in the windows as the cork is eased from a bottle of champagne for the traditional wetting of the baby's head.

Dennis offers us a glass and we both shake our heads.

'Drat.' We grin at one another.

Leonie produces the birth-day cake and we all bask in gratitude for the little one's safe arrival. In the middle of it all, there is yet another knock on the door.

It is Cathy's neighbour.

'Did you get your car going?' Ivan asks.

'Unfortunately, no.' She shrugs. 'Had to walk, but a lovely morning for it.'

—⁜—

'Adele, it's Cathy. It's all on! My waters have broken, and the contractions have started and become more regular.'

It is two years on, now. Cathy's boy is a robust two-year-old, and she is about to have another baby.

After she finishes talking to Cathy, Adele phones Leonie. It is 8 pm, but we can do this now. The old manual telephone exchange system has been replaced by the same automated system that practically everyone else in New Zealand has been enjoying for some time.

'Cathy has started contracting,' she says. 'I'm heading off shortly.'

'I don't think you should go,' Leonie says. 'You need to look after yourself. That's the most important thing, Adele. Why don't you stay home?'

'No, I can manage,' Adele says. 'I told Cathy that I would be there. She's relying on me.'

'You need to look after yourself,' Leonie reiterates.

'Actually,' Adele begins, then stops. She struggles to control her voice. 'Actually, I would rather have something to do. I can cope. I'll have to.'

There is a long silence.

'OK. I'll come with Ivan, then,' Leonie says. 'We'll see you there.'

The concern and empathy in her voice nearly starts Adele crying again. But after she has hung up the phone she gathers her gear. The familiar routine steadies her. She loads the car, gets in, takes a deep breath and sets off.

Leonie's mum is staying with them, as she has been doing every summer since first Amiria and then Jordan were born. Summer is a crazy time: the resident population is swamped by an influx of holidaymakers, and Ivan and Leonie would be busy enough without being the parents of two small children and their older brother, Alastair. Jordan is just five and a half months and still breastfeeding. The rising tide of their belongings is an indicator that there is also a busy, enquiring two-year-old Amiria about. Alastair is currently sprawled on the couch, absorbed in a book.

Leonie rushes about gathering gear as her mum helps by ticking items off on a checklist. Leonie had not been counting on attending this birth as a midwife due to Jordan's needs, but she wants to support Adele. Her mum straps a sleepy baby into his car seat, as they carry the midwifery gear and the baby gear out to the car. Jordan simply smiles drowsily. Leonie and Ivan set off on the familiar twenty-minute drive to Cathy and Dennis's new house in the Tryphena bush.

The roads rock Jordan back to sleep.

'I don't think we should take him inside,' Ivan says. 'We don't want him waking up and distracting Cathy in the middle of the birth. Let's leave him in his car seat. We can park the car right up by the window so we can see him if he wakes up.'

Leonie is happy with this arrangement, so Ivan and Dennis start manoeuvring vehicles so that their own is just 30 centimetres from the window of the room where Cathy is. Leonie takes her gear inside.

There to greet her are Cathy, who smiles, flushed and dishevelled— the labour is progressing quickly—and Nancy, whom Adele has asked to attend until Leonie arrives, in case Cathy's birth is fast.

Leonie can see Jordan through the window of the room and the window of the car. It is a grandstand view. The light spilling from the room lights his face as he sleeps.

Cathy is feeling the contractions intensely now. Similar to last time, she is positioned on a mattress on the floor. She is bundled up in Dennis's Swanndri and breathing hard through each contraction. Leonie listens to the baby and is reassured by the regular heartbeat that all is well. Leonie believes Cathy is in transition, and that the birth is imminent.

Cathy is very pale. 'I think I need to push now,' she pants.

With several pushes and a soft groan or two, a big baby girl slips into the world. Her colour is slightly dusky and she is a little floppy, which is a cause for concern. But, as she lies on Cathy's chest, she quickly pinks up, and her heart and lungs sound normal. Cathy lies back, shocked and shaking with the speed of it. But after a few minutes, sipping the hot drink that Nancy brings her, her own colour is returning too.

Leonie sneaks a look out of the window. Jordan is still sleeping peacefully.

Lights shine up the drive and a car arrives. It's Adele. She enters the room with a sad smile.

Leonie makes sure that Adele sits in an armchair and watches as the placenta is delivered. It is intact, and all seems normal. It is time for Leonie to clean up and to present her customary birth-day cake, and for Dennis to open the bottle of champagne. Cathy proudly announces her ten-pound daughter's name.

'Johanna. Her name's meaning is Gift of God in Hebrew,' says Ivan.

Leonie checks on Jordan, and then turns her attention to Adele.

We share a long, strong hug. The significance escapes everyone but Ivan.

After eighteen years of marriage, Adele got some aspect of her family planning wrong. She was initially devastated when, a couple of months before, she had looked at the pregnancy test and it read positive. However, she and Shannon eventually talked themselves around to accepting the situation, and even looked forward to being parents—which is why this has been one of the hardest afternoons in her life. The symptoms of the pregnancy, which had been very strong, had slackened over the last couple of days, and all doubt vanished earlier this afternoon when Adele started cramping. At 4 pm, she miscarried.

We had talked on the phone several times—both of us crying—before Cathy's call came. Leonie had been trying to persuade Adele to take some leave off-island and, at the very least, to let Nancy, Ivan and Leonie attend Cathy's birth, when it happened. But Adele was adamant that she would be there for Cathy, as promised.

Leonie had hung up from the last call feeling a terrible, impotent grief for her friend and something resembling guilt at the joy she had in her own two happy, healthy children. But during the hour-long drive from Port FitzRoy to Tryphena, Adele had time to reflect. It was all part of it, she knew. The same circle of renewal that saw her making this drive the length of the island again for Cathy was the cycle that had both given and taken away her own pregnancy. Death is part of life.

Now, in this room filled with Cathy and Dennis's joy, with Leonie stealing glances out of the window at the angelic, softly lit features of her sleeping baby, Adele feels a kind of peace. She thinks about one of her patients, an older Aotea resident, who told her about the series of miscarriages she suffered at a time when such things were not spoken about. She feels a deep empathy for that woman, and all women who have had to bear such grief alone. She is thankful that she will be supported in her loss in the same way and by the same community as Cathy and the other mothers of Aotea are supported in the joyful delivery of their infants, and that thought is an immense comfort to her.

That weekend, Adele sits in the quiet of her home and stitches together a quilt for Cathy's new baby girl. As she does so, she celebrates the strength of women and the bonds that are created in shared birth experiences and of the miracle that is childbirth. She thinks with love about the baby. As her needle passes in and out of the fabric, she smiles through her tears.

Chapter 7

ONWARDS, UPWARDS

One of the stories that highlighted how badly change was needed didn't happen to us; it was Nancy who was in the hot seat. It was on one of the rare occasions when Leonie and Ivan were off-island. They seldom went away because it was no easy task getting a general practitioner to come and locum, working from the caravan. Nancy clearly recalls the chain of events.

One starry night, she got a call from the very worried wife of a 40-year-old local man. He had, she said, a 'sore stomach'.

Knowing the couple well, Nancy knew they wouldn't be calling her unless it was serious. Nancy's instincts were to attend immediately.

She moved her vehicle as close as she could to the man's house, parking her small four-wheel-drive at the bottom of the steep, winding track that was the only access. She made the ascent by torchlight, and arrived to find a very worried woman hovering at the door.

Her husband was pale and sweaty and clearly in agony, and had been vomiting brownish, granular material for hours. Nancy gave him a quick examination, and found his blood pressure to be low and his pulse fast and thready. It supported what she already suspected: he was probably bleeding from a stomach ulcer. The 'coffee grounds' that he had been vomiting were altered blood—blood affected by gastric juices. He urgently needed to be transferred to Auckland Hospital. She cranked up the phone and asked the operator for Auckland Hospital so as to facilitate a speedy admission. It took a while, but eventually she was connected with a doctor who was prepared to accept a rural nurse's diagnosis and to authorise admission.

Nancy's relief was short-lived.

No sooner had she put down the phone than her thoughts suddenly turned to the steep track to the road. She surveyed her patient: he was a big man, and the combined strength of his wife and she, the not-so-young nurse, was never going to be enough to get him down it.

That was the first thing that struck her. The second was that, while she knew it was vital that he be administered fluids to replace the volume he had lost through vomiting in order to stabilise his condition, she had never inserted an intravenous line before.

Nancy felt pretty alone at this point.

Priorities, she thought. She inserted the line by the wavering light of a torch as though she had been doing it all her life, and soon she had normal saline snaking into his vein from a bag his wife was holding aloft.

Now it was time to address the evacuation issue. She needed to find at least four strong men, and it was early in the night. When she cranked up the phone again to ask the sleepy local operator if he could rustle up some help for her, the best he could come up with was a contingent from the local Barrier Social Club.

Time was of the essence, she thought. Great Barrier Airlines were already preparing for take-off from Auckland.

Loud crashing and the odd giggle announced the arrival of her stretcher-bearers. Three short figures from the club and one tall neighbour emerged from the inky blackness at the top of the track. They had the scoop stretcher from Nancy's car with them, and the patient was soon secured on it with straps around his torso and the blanket tucked tightly around his legs. With Nancy holding the IV line aloft, and when all seemed in order, the bearers hoisted the stretcher. With one much taller than the other three and (it became clear) one of them pretty inebriated, Nancy could tell the patient, even in his distress, thought it was odds-on he would be tobogganing most of the way down the hillside.

With Nancy following and shining her torch on the IV line, which she was sure would be ripped out somewhere en route, the party set off. The track switched to and fro down the hillside. The patient swore at regular intervals and, despite being well strapped in, gripped the sides of the stretcher with white knuckles.

Somehow, they made it to the road without mishap. Another volunteer had opened the tailgate of Nancy's four-wheel-drive and had been struggling manfully with the mechanism that reclined the seat backs. He thought they were jammed. There was no way the stretcher would fit in the interior without being able to lie the seats flat.

The locals scratched their heads and mulled over the options. Eventually, someone had the bright idea of fetching the school bus. Someone jogged off to rouse the driver.

Everyone stood about for a few minutes, with Nancy checking her patient. Then the sound of a diesel motor could be heard and headlights splashed across the canopy of the trees. The elderly school bus hauled into view. It crawled past the group, stopped and then the reversing siren started and the patient on his stretcher was lit in the ghostly glow of the reversing lamps. The driver clearly aimed to get as close as he could to spare the patient as much discomfort as possible.

Everyone watched for a moment, chatting idly. Then the conversation stopped and there was a flurry of anxiety.

'Stop! Stop!' several people frantically yelled, including the patient himself, immobilised and watching the wheels on the bus going round and round and ever nearer.

The bus jerked to a halt.

As soon as the doors hissed open, someone realised that the stretcher was wider than the aisle between the seats. Another committee meeting was convened to decide where to put the stretcher, and it was finally decided to secure it across the top of the seats. Nancy had visions of emergency braking, the stretcher launched through the windscreen like a missile . . . But there was no time to devise better arrangements, and soon the bus roared off over the metal roads, drip miraculously still intact, on its way to the airfield, 30 minutes away. Nurse Nancy was much relieved.

Evacuation from the airstrip at night, in the late 1980s, was still very much dependant on a fixed-wing plane and local support people. Only the most experienced commercial pilots were permitted to fly to the Barrier by night, and even then the Civil Aviation Authority limited this to emergency evacuations for patients who could not be left until daylight. The grass airstrip was unlit, so locals were roused or gathered from the local clubs to provide runway lighting. Strategic cars would park along the runway with their headlights on. One night—it may even have been that night, since it was that sort of night—on the instructions of a new policeman who thought his grid layout to be an improvement, the cars were duly arranged. The locals, not wanting to disappoint him, obliged, only to hear the plane circling above instead of landing. Everyone looked at everyone else and wondered what the problem was.

Soon afterward, a car arrived at speed. It was the Tryphena telephone operator, who had been woken by Great Barrier Airlines ground control instructing him to race over the hill and get the clowns whose lights were dazzling the pilot on his approach to turn in the opposite direction. The Claris exchange was closed, and this was long before cell phones. Orders were issued and cars rearranged—to reveal a lone car, headlights off, in the centre of the runway. An urgent investigation revealed that the driver was fast asleep in his seat.

It is amazing what you get used to, and what you can come to consider normal. Leonie and Ivan managed to find a bigger, racier, more modern caravan than the green one, although their new orange one was still pretty elderly. Leonie politely asked Ivan that it be sited further from their front door and closer to the roadway, to give everyone—both them and their patients—a modicum of privacy when they had visitors. So, Ivan and his assistants wheeled the new caravan to and fro with much grunting and studying of angles. When they thought they had it organised, they chocked the wheels and boxed it in to stay. Leonie was pleased with the new position, at first. The shortcomings only became obvious to her the first time she was performing a well-woman check (she had begun to offer cervical smears and antenatal checks as part of her evolving nursing-midwifery role) and she heard male voices. Ivan had intercepted their next patient at the front gate and had detained him there, chatting, while Leonie knelt, torch angled, performing a gynaecological examination. Although the new caravan was bigger, it still only had a narrow bunk on either side of a cramped aisle: the poor female patient had to lie on the bunk, legs spread, while Leonie knelt in the aisle. If someone were to open the locked door, there was no way anyone could retain their dignity, let alone their modesty.

Everything professional seemed to be a struggle. The culture on the island is very much one of making do, as it has to be. We simply had to follow the islanders' lead with what we could provide. Nevertheless, it seemed wrong to be offering such a third-world service only 30 minutes' flight from the modernity of Auckland.

One night, after they had been in their larger caravan for a while, Ivan and Leonie had an emergency. A man had been brought to them unconscious and Ivan, on his hands and knees on the caravan floor with a torch in his mouth, was trying to secure the patient's airway using first an oropharyngeal airway (a short tube that is fed from the mouth into the patient's windpipe) and then connecting this to an Ambu bag (which can be used to manually ventilate a patient who is not breathing adequately for themselves). Leonie knew what he was trying to communicate around the torch, even though the words were unintelligible: he wanted an extra pair of hands. The trouble was, with both Ivan and the island's solid policeman crowded in the space around the patient, there was simply no room for Leonie to assist.

Somehow, Ivan got the patient intubated and organised for evacuation. After he had been sent off on the plane, Ivan put his head in his hands and said, 'I can't do this anymore—the community deserves better.'

He and Leonie talked it over. The problem was that neither local nor central government could be persuaded to take responsibility for providing facilities for what was, in effect, a private medical practice.

Other remote areas in New Zealand had been made 'Special Areas' by the Ministry of Health, where the health service was free to the community. Great Barrier Island, unfortunately, remained the square peg that would not fit into the round holes of the funding models. The Great Barrier Island County Council with its small rateable base could not afford to build a facility like many other rural New Zealand local bodies had been able to do.

'We could leave,' Ivan suggested. 'If we left, they would have to take responsibility.'

'Where would we go?'

Ivan considered it. 'China, perhaps?' he mused.

He had been born to medical missionary parents in Yantai, in China's north-eastern Shandong province. A few years before, he and his sister had returned there for a school reunion, and he told Leonie it was as though he had gone home. He could imagine them living and working there.

But Leonie looked around their little house thoughtfully. It did not feel as though the Howies were finished with Aotea quite yet.

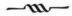

It wasn't just us who could see the value of a properly equipped medical clinic. The islanders had already reached the same conclusion. Fortunately, some of the locals were doing a bit of research of their own.

One day in the late eighties, Ivan rushed through the front door, beaming.

'Helen suggests I speak with the local council about a community health centre,' he told Leonie. 'She's been looking at the district plan, and there's a clause in there about the need for a medical centre. She is sure the islanders will find a creative solution!'

Helen O'Shea was a former psychiatric nurse who had moved with her husband to the Awana Valley on the Barrier to become farmers. Although she once described herself as 'the president of the newcomers' club', she had been on the island nearly twenty years by the time she was elected to the County Council. Her rural outlook typified most Barrierites—with twinkling eyes and smile set in a broad face beneath her curly auburn hair, she was unfailingly optimistic and possessed of apparently boundless, indomitable energy. Firmly believing that there had to be a better way to arrange things medical on Aotea, she had dug out the 42-year-old district plan and found, to her delight, that those drafting it had declared their intention 'to investigate the possibility of establishing a medical centre in Claris'. A precedent had been set. If there had been a perceived need nearly half a century ago, Helen argued, how much more necessary was a medical centre now? She encouraged Ivan to attend a meeting of the County Council to put the case forward.

So while Leonie 'held the fort'—that is, stayed handy to their telephone in case an emergency call came—Ivan, Adele and Nancy met the county councillors. The fact that their predecessors had identified a need for a medical centre was news to the councillors, but with Helen fired up about the issue, they were relatively easily persuaded to agree in principle to find a solution for Aotea's health infrastructure problems.

While Ivan and Adele were buoyed by this development, Leonie wasn't so sure. She could see the enormous amount of money that would be needed, and she wondered how a community so impecunious would ever find the funds necessary to construct a medical centre by itself.

For a while, it seemed she was right. After the initial buzz from the meeting had worn off, hope dwindled and nothing happened. Ivan and Leonie went right back to kneeling in the caravan to examine their patients, and the need to get on with it swamped any such thoughts of a medical centre: they were busy, as before, just staying afloat.

Helen was not to be deterred, however. She persuaded the County Council to create a committee comprising volunteers along with the health professionals: each of the geographical regions (north, central, south) were represented, as were the tangata whenua, and there was a broad range of opinion and expertise aboard as well. This 'health committee' met regularly, and at some point the notion of a Community Health Trust evolved—ensuring that the ownership of the health infrastructure would remain firmly with the community. Ivan and Leonie were particularly in favour of this: it meant that if death or disaster befell them or their practice, all that would be needed would be for new health practitioners to step in, future-proofing the service. The islanders need not notice any change in the health service. Besides, the community's sense of identity being as it is, making the health system the islanders' own would be far more than merely symbolic.

David Palmer, a local with some experience with trusts, was duly enlisted to draft a Trust Deed, and in June 1988, the inaugural trustees of the Great Barrier Island Community Health Trust set their signatures to it. Helen O'Shea made short work of the bureaucratic difficulties that attend becoming a charitable organisation. We had the structure in place; now it was the not-so-simple matter of raising the funds to make the dream a reality.

Ironically, the first donation the trust ever received came from a home-brew competition that was held in the Tryphena Hall directly after the Alcoholics Anonymous meeting had been ushered out. Everyone wanted to be involved—there were birdman competitions where locals dressed as birds and flung themselves off Tryphena wharf to cheers and jeers. There were Irish stews and raffles. A ratepayers' grant of $10,000 from Great Barrier Island County Council consolidated the seeding fund; a bequest from an older, much-esteemed resident completed it. Over $30,000 would have been a tall order at any time for a community such as the Barrier's, but to have amassed that total in just two years in the straitened economic climate that prevailed at the end of the 1980s was little short of miraculous.

Meanwhile, Ivan had been networking on the mainland. The real turning point in the trust's fortunes came courtesy of Dame Cath Tizard, who at that time was the Mayor of Auckland City and was also on the ASB Community Trust. Dame Cath was very sympathetic to Ivan's request for support. One day, she arrived on the island waving a huge cheque from the ASB Community Trust. She joyfully painted in the top of the red fundraising thermometer, indicating that our goal had been reached at last. The grant was enormous, and it was enough to build the long dreamed-of community health centre.

As if that weren't good enough news, the same meeting that was convened to formally accept the ASB Community Trust grant also heard that the Auckland Area Health Board had offered to donate a four-bedroom state house from the old Carrington Hospital to our cause. It took the trustees all of five minutes to decide to accept both.

Hang on. Was it possible to accept both? Enquiries were made, and we were assured it most definitely was possible. The money from the ASB Community Trust could be used to redesign and outfit the Carrington building—expanding the original concept.

Anyone standing on the white sands of Kaitoke Beach on the morning of 8 January 1990—and there was quite a crowd of us— would have found the sight of the little weatherboard house, painted cream and lemon with an orange tile roof, chugging around the point in the lee of the humped island just offshore quite surreal. The barge was manoeuvred into the surf where a bulldozer was waiting to attach a long yoke to the hydraulic trailer on which the building rested. The trailer, house and all, was dragged off and hauled up the beach. There was a pause while one of the locals, just to be sure, inspected the building to make sure nothing had stowed away inside. Good job he did: he found two possums hiding in the roof space. Because it is just far enough from the mainland, Great Barrier has always been free of possums. The beach was cleared of people. The policeman fetched his revolver, there were two sharp cracks and Aotea was possum free again. The border biosecurity formalities over, the bulldozer's engine bellowed and the house was dragged up the sandy track through the dunes to the site close to the airfield, where it was to be transformed into the Great Barrier Island Community Health Trust's new community health centre.

Over the previous two years, while the funds were being raised, a lot of thought had gone into how the health centre should be configured. Gale Gibson, a trustee who worked for Barrier Building, had a great relationship with all of the local tradespeople and plenty more on the mainland, enabling him access to valuable information and ideas. The renovation and modification of the building was a truly collaborative effort: the local island architect did a superb job of the design, creating a multifunctional community health centre with the added funds; and the efforts of other skilled contractors, led by Lance Dixon—builders, plumbers, electrician, painters and cabinetmakers, all of them locals—soon saw it clad in new cedar and running on alternative energy, using thousands of dollars' worth of donated materials. Up to 58 different mainland companies or persons supported the trust, too, to realise the islanders' dream. Locals donated voluntary hours and expertise, an amazing stone sculpture depicting strength in unity and family, art pieces, crotchet rugs, linen and aroha nui. Helen and her team were there every step of the way.

We already had modern equipment that had been donated lined up to install. We would no longer need to hang bags of intravenous fluid from a nail at the top of a mānuka pole while we waited in someone's car for the plane to land; we could be in a warm, cosy, well-lit room right beside the airfield with the drip suspended from a stainless-steel IV stand with proper wheels. There was an overnight room with two comfortable beds where people could be cared for. There was a steriliser, a sterile area for minor surgery, an organised daily appointment system and, one day very soon, there would be an X-ray machine. It even had a brand-new automated telephone—the advent of the automated system coincided with the establishment of the health centre. Imagine that—being able to pick up the phone and talk to the hospital, any time of the day or night, without having to worry about confidentiality on the line or the need to drive anywhere to wake an operator!

On Labour Weekend 1990, the Governor-General, Sir Paul Reeves, emerged from a Royal New Zealand Airforce Iroquois helicopter and was escorted across the airfield to where a crowd was waiting for the formal opening of our new community health centre.

There were speeches, and lots of laughter and excitement. The community were justly proud of what they had achieved: there could be no doubt that this was progress.

Adele spoke, and she spoke for island nurses past and present.

'To me, this building epitomises the things that I find very special about Great Barrier Island—the sense of community spirit, resourcefulness and determination that its residents possess. Nursing has to do with caring for people, and it was with absolute amazement that I discovered in this community the reverse also applied, in that the nurses were also cared for and valued by the people. Thinking about the special affinity that the island has had with its nurses and looking up at this modern building demonstrates to me the importance the community places upon health.'

Sir Paul spoke, and then cut the ribbon. Helen grabbed Ivan's hand and shook it. 'Congratulations!' She beamed. 'We did it! The islanders have prevailed!'

The Great Barrier Island medical facilities had finally leaped towards the twenty-first century.

With the health centre up and running, there was one last duty for the Howies to perform. Ivan and Leonie watched as the orange caravan was hauled away on flat tyres and in a cloud of dust. They hugged. It was the end of an era, and, while it had been a strange way to operate a medical practice, it was also somehow picturesque. Leonie was surprised at the sadness she felt.

But on her very first day in the brand-new clinic her sadness is gone. It is as though she has been travelling towards her professional destination these last few years, and has only just arrived. The clinic feels right, and somehow validates her.

The phone rings, and she answers. She hears the change in her voice, and so does the local on the other end. It is not the doctor's wife answering. It is Leonie, the rural nurse.

We had seen a kind of tidal ebb and flow in the former days of the Department of Health. Sometimes the people in decision-making positions understood the demands and requirements of rural nursing. Sometimes they seemed to think that it was little different to working in a well-stocked clinic in a leafy suburb with straightforward access to all main transport modes and all medical mod cons.

The vehicles that Adele and Nancy were finally supplied with reflected the degree to which the urban managers misunderstood what it meant to try to supply health services to the sparse population on a mountainous island with a very poor roading system. Adele's first Health Board vehicle was a Toyota Land Cruiser (Nancy had a four-wheel-drive Suzuki). But when the time came to replace them, there had been a change in personnel in the vehicle procurement department. It was decided that Nancy should have a station wagon and they sent Adele a boxy little two-door four-wheel-drive Lada. Nancy did what she could with the station wagon, but island conditions took their toll upon it. When it went back to Auckland full of dust and with all the doors rattling, Nancy was accused of not caring for it.

Adele's Lada stood up to the rigours of the roading rather better, but she couldn't fit her patients in it, and it was so poorly designed that she developed a repetitive strain injury in her left shoulder from the difficult gear changes. She grew to loathe the vehicle. But the day was at hand when she could get shot of it, and ensure that its replacement was much more fit for purpose.

In 1992, Adele and Shannon attended a one-week intensive small-business course that was run on the island by the Auckland New Venture Trust. They had finally got their mussel-farming venture off the ground, and the course introduced them to some of the processes needed to operate a small business—such as wrangling taxes like PAYE and GST, and how to write a business plan. Ivan and Leonie were there too, as their medical practice was growing fast. Little did we all know that we would be using the skills we acquired to take Great Barrier's health services another quantum leap forward.

In July 1993, New Zealand's health system was radically reformed.

Funding and procurement was shifted from the Department of Health, which was renamed the Ministry of Health, to newly formed Regional Health Authorities (RHAs). The management of the Northern RHA (North Health) was largely in the hands of people who wished to improve health-service delivery and reduce costs, and, consequently, they were far more receptive to suggestions for new and better ways of providing services. We all immediately saw the opportunity that the brave new funding model presented. It might mean that we could finally set up a comprehensive health service tailored specifically to meet the needs of the people of Aotea.

So together we wrote a business plan, describing the community's health needs—rated as 'remote rural' in the official classification system—and proposed a new organisation to cater efficiently to these needs and to accommodate the unique demands that the island imposed. The new enterprise would pool the public and private revenue streams, and we would combine the expertise of the private practitioners with that of the public health nurses and engage additional professionals to provide a comprehensive health service. Our proposal was supported by Dr John McLeod (CEO of the Auckland RHA) and his deputy, Dr Colin Tukuitonga. John had been Medical Officer of Health and in this role had made regular visits to the island and had met with Adele, as public health nurse, and with Ivan and Leonie. John saw for himself the extent of Ivan's dedication to the island. He had also watched with interest the formation and achievements of the Great Barrier Island Community Health Trust, and he could see that our proposal was the logical next step.

Aotea Health Limited was duly incorporated on 2 August 1994. Ivan designed the company logo—an elegant motif that at once resembles a Māori design and also a stylised map of Aotea itself. We are the directors. We have ended up working to our strengths, with

Adele doing the finances and Leonie island-proofing the policies, and both of us sharing everything else along with full-time clinical work. For his part, Ivan liked the idea of being a doctor free from the burden of running the business and getting mixed up in the fine details of contracts. Within days of launching the company, Adele had resigned from her position as public health nurse. She took great pleasure in sending the Lada back to the mainland. She has often joked since that it was the Lada that convinced her to enter private enterprise.

The first task ahead of our new venture was negotiating with the service funders. On the one hand, it was a refreshing change to deal directly with those holding the purse strings, instead of having to go through an intermediary. On the other hand, it turned out that it came with its own unique range of frustrations and was never plain sailing.

Adele sat on the floor surrounded by paper—the draft of a contract that we had agreed with the RHA and a newer, final version that had just spooled from the fax machine. They were more or less the same—apart from the sum the RHA was now offering to pay for our services, which was mysteriously $20,000 less than the agreed figure.

What? Adele wondered. *Did they think we wouldn't notice?*

She phoned the funding manager, but his receptionist told her he would not take her call. Adele felt close to tears. She checked her watch. Ivan and Leonie were on their way off-island for a two-week holiday. Here she was, unemployed and confronted with a contract that would doom the fledgling new enterprise to failure.

Adele phoned the airport. The airline agreed to hold the plane and to fetch Ivan off it. After a delay, Ivan came on the line. She explained the situation.

'But that's not what we agreed,' Ivan said. 'I will try to ring as well.'

Adele waited on tenterhooks. The phone rang.

'He agreed to change the figure back,' Ivan said. 'He will fax us a guarantee that we'll get the missing funds.'

Adele heaved a sigh of relief mixed with irony that Ivan had managed to get through.

Sure enough, the fax came to life and a document on North Health letterhead slowly emerged. It was a written guarantee. Crisis averted, and lesson learned: inspect every version of a contract with a fine-tooth comb! When we compared notes on the whole experience later, we also agreed that we needed to have a backup plan in place in future, to say nothing of strategies by which to navigate tortuous health-funding hierarchies that didn't know us.

That experience was a one-off, but that is not to say that the funding rounds were plain sailing. There were endless bureaucratic changes between 1993 and 1999 that posed challenges. With each new structural change, it seemed a new set of managers came aboard who had little understanding of island health service issues. Fortunately, the RHA senior echelon remained very supportive, and this consolidated our position.

One funding round we were summoned to Auckland to attend a meeting. We had not budgeted for trips to Auckland and the expense that this would put us to. It so happened that for Aotea Health the management staff were also the clinical staff. We would need to hire a locum doctor and nurses—at our own considerable expense.

Still, we made the trip, and on our way it occurred to us that this was the first time we three had all been off the island at the same time. It was quite exciting, especially since it gave us an opportunity to do nothing but focus on the business.

Two hours before we were supposed to leave the place where we were staying for the drive to the meeting, a call came on Adele's cell phone. She fumbled with it—this was all new to her—and answered.

'They want to postpone,' she said.

'What? Why? Until when?'

'They didn't say. There was no explanation.'

We were in a tricky position. The longer we stayed in Auckland, the more it would cost us all to stay there and to pay for locums to minimise the disruption to the operation of our business. Should we stay or should we go?

Adele phoned anyone she could think of who might have influence over the funding organisation, and eventually managed to get a commitment that the meeting would take place the next day.

So the following morning we parked directly outside the offices of the funder. A receptionist looked up from her desk as we entered.

'You can't park there,' she said briskly. 'You'll be towed.'

We reshuffled the rental car into a safe park. Then, after a wait, we were admitted to the meeting room. We were all expecting the assembled managers to be conciliatory, or at least apologetic for the unexplained delay and the inconvenience to which it had put us.

'First, Ms Robertson, I'd like to say that I didn't appreciate being rung when I was on sick leave to be pressured about this meeting,' the funding manager said tartly.

'Well, we have expended a considerable amount of time and money to come to this meeting,' Ivan replied hotly. 'And we did not appreciate being left adrift in Auckland, not knowing whether to return to the island or not. I would also like to say that your receptionist was rude.'

'Ivan,' Leonie soothed, but Adele was agreeing with him. He was saying exactly what she was feeling.

'No, this is outrageous,' Ivan said. 'This whole experience isn't what we would have expected from an organisation responsible for health.'

There was silence. Everyone stared at everyone else.

'I think we should start again,' Leonie suggested. 'We'll go out and come back in and we'll try again.'

So that is what we did. It was another valuable learning experience for us—in future, we would try to hold all funding meetings on the island so that the funders could experience for themselves the cost of travel, the vagaries of plane and ferry schedules disrupted by weather, and the time it cost you when that happened. It would also let them see us in our own professional environment, where the spirit of Aotea seems to get in the room so that meetings are run in a warm and constructive manner.

One sobering fact we learned during the business course we attended in 1992 was that many small businesses fail in their first few years. We decided that, from the outset, we needed to be very hands-on, especially with finances. After the fiasco with the missing $20,000, we never again fully trusted that the promised funds would come through until they actually arrived in our bank account so, like most small business owners when the going is tough, we reduced our salaries so we would always have a float for a rainy day.

To this day, staff salaries are our biggest expense. Our vision was to employ rural nurses and experienced GPs to provide a wide range of services to a defined population for a fixed price. We felt we had sold this concept to the RHA senior echelon, but then it was handed over to the managers, who wanted us to divide the money into separate contracts for seven different speciality areas of healthcare. In the end, we randomly assigned figures to each of the contracts so that it all added up to the total amount agreed upon. As a result, we hold multiple contracts but, given the nature of the work on Great Barrier, we can be working across all of them on any given day.

Teething troubles and the occasional glitch aside, the system has worked. In 2014, the Auckland District Health Board (as it is now termed) conducted a series of community meetings to solicit community input into the services that Aotea Health provide. The feedback was overwhelmingly that the community has an excellent service and that the ADHB should do all that they can to support it—which they have done.

Adele was at one of these meetings when the Auckland DHB organisers asked if there were any problems with alcohol abuse in the community. Around the table were several faces bearing the sadness of those who grow up in families affected by alcohol.

This will be interesting, she thought.

'No,' someone said at length. 'No. We don't have alcohol issues.'

Adele suppressed a smile. Afterwards, as they were washing the dishes from the meeting in the kitchen attached to the hall, she found herself alongside the spokesperson on the issue.

'So,' she said, 'what's the story with no alcohol issues?'

'No way was I going to air our dirty laundry in front of a bunch of strangers, Adele,' came the answer.

Adele nodded and thought that the reply got to the heart of rural nursing: the 'insider' relationship built over time on trust was important.

Chapter 8

ANSWERING THE CALL

Among the many and various qualities you need as a rural nurse is versatility: the ability to have the knowledge and skills to answer any call. This also involves having the ability to understand your patients' needs because of your knowledge of their community, of their context. We are obliged to be generalists in order to perform within what is technically called our broad scope of practice. In our role, we therefore have a little knowledge about the wide spectrum of illness and trauma pathology that we may encounter during our day-to-day practice. But, every now and again, we are reminded that the inverse is also true. There is a lot we *don't* know about some of the more specialist nursing skills. Nurse generalism versus specialism expresses the tension between the breadth of knowledge and the depth of knowledge a rural nurse needs to have.

There is a knock, quiet but urgent, on the back door of the nurse's station at the health centre. Leonie opens it and is surprised to find a young woman whom she knows well—usually of warm and smiling disposition, and totally in control of situations—looking pale, shocked and plainly on the verge of tears.

'It's Hemi,' she says. 'He's had an accident.'

Hemi* is bundled into the relative warmth of the clinic with a bloody towel pressed to the left side of his face. He is dressed in a wetsuit.

Leonie and Hemi's partner help him on to the examination couch.

'What have you done?' Leonie asks.

'Wiped out. The sharp point of my surfboard slammed into my eye socket,' he says, his voice tight with pain. Tears are welling within his partner's eyes, although Leonie can see she is desperately trying to be staunch for Hemi's sake.

Leonie takes a brief history, and checks his vital signs. Hemi is 26 and otherwise very fit and healthy. On examination, she finds him hypothermic (cold), bradycardic (slow pulse) and hypotensive (low blood pressure). He seems to have normal vision in his right eye on cursory examination, and when she checks him for possible brain injuries she finds him conscious with no other obvious signs of an internal head injury.

'I'm going to need to quickly have a look at the eye so that we can see what we are dealing with,' she tells him. 'Then we can give you something for the pain.'

She scrubs up and pulls on a pair of gloves, and then he removes the towel he is still holding clamped to his face. There is a puncture

---

* Not his real name.

wound on his cheek a little below his left eye, and there are a couple of obvious minor lacerations closer to the eye itself. When she gently raises the lid of the eye itself, she finds the eye socket filled with a thrombus (a blood clot) masking any internal structures.

This is all clearly major, and well outside Leonie's expertise. She hastily applies a light dressing comprising a saline-soaked gauze pad to the eye, and then calls Ivan to discuss a plan.

He listens to her description of the injury

'I'll get there as quick as I can,' he says. 'But, in the meantime, you will need to get his pain under control.'

He offers specific instructions on the analgesia to administer. Between herself and his partner, they wrestle Hemi out of his wetsuit. As soon as she has access to his arm, Leonie gives him some pain relief intravenously and an anti-emetic to prevent nausea: the last thing a damaged eye needs is the pressure that vomiting causes. They bundle him up in woollen blankets—enough to warm him, but not so much that he will overheat.

Ivan arrives. He wastes no time in scrubbing up so that he can perform a detailed examination. As he removes the thrombus, he remarks that, contrary to popular belief, the eye wall is strong and will often survive a blow administered with great force.

But as soon as he begins his inspection any optimism he might have felt leaves him.

'It's not good, I'm afraid,' he says. 'I can see most of the very inner structures of the eye.'

Now that the pain relief is working, Hemi seems more curious about his injury than anything else.

'What can you see?' he asks.

'Well, I can see some of your inner eye soggily clinging to your lower eyelid. The sclera has been badly damaged . . .'

Hemi continues to ask questions while Leonie phones the Auckland Hospital Eye Registrar to discuss Hemi's pending admission and then to request the despatch of the Auckland Rescue Helicopter. Hemi naturally wants to know what his chances of being able to see out of that eye are. Ivan deflects those questions. It is not until after he gets to the Eye Department at Auckland Hospital an hour later, and undergoes an examination under general anaesthetic that Hemi is told his chances of regaining sight in his left eye are pretty much nil.

Hemi has always loved surfing. He has described it to Leonie as 'riding on God's energy'. He was surfing a break at a remote Aotea beach that beautiful spring day when the wave broke and pitched him, board and all, into the water. The nose of his board struck him directly in his left eye and the weight of the water pressed him down into the sand. It took all his reserves, as he will tell Leonie later, to stay conscious and to fight his way back to the surface. He remembers that first gasp of air as the sweetest of his life.

He doesn't remember much about the struggle up the track from the beach, or the 40-minute drive to the health centre. It all has the quality of a nightmare from which he has been unable to wake.

The hospital performs a basic repair soon after admission. Later, one of the specialist eye nurses explains to Leonie that it is standard procedure in cases of major trauma to the eye: as the swelling subsides over the course of the next few days, the patient can come to terms with their loss before actual enucleation (the removal of the eye) is performed.

The CT scan shows that there are blowout fractures in the eye socket floor with soft tissue prolapsing into the adjacent sinus. It seems that the nose of the surfboard entered his eye socket directly and destroyed the eye; another millimetre or so and it would likely have entered his brain.

While he is resting in his hospital bed with both eyes bandaged, Hemi is in a dream-like state, a place where, as he tells Leonie, time both stands still and moves at a million miles per hour. It is hard to get a grasp on what is real and what is imaginary. The eye nurses indicated to Leonie the importance of voice and touch in providing comfort and reassurance when one's world is tipped on its axis. They are an anchor in the confusion. It is a reassurance that he is still alive, and this is something that he clings to.

Ten days after admission, the eye is removed and the socket reconstructed, the preliminary step before fitting Hemi with an ocular prosthesis (a false eye) down the track.

Hemi's whakapapa is Ngāti Kikopiri, a hapū of the Ngāti Raukawa iwi. His cultural heritage is rich with Māori and Pākehā kinship ties, and he moves easily between both cultures—but, as he recovers from his injury, he tells Leonie that perhaps because of his bushman grandfather, who was a big influence upon him as he was growing up, it is from his Māori heritage that he draws strength and the necessary perspective to deal with grief and loss.

Eventually he, his partner and their child can return to Aotea to continue his rehabilitation. Leonie has followed his progress every step of the way. The eye nurses hand over to her to supervise the ongoing process. She has admired their specialised skills, and appreciates their advice in how to support Hemi in his recovery. He is still experiencing throbbing pain in the eye socket. Sometimes it is in the background; other times it is severe. He is also bothered by dizziness. The eye nurses assure Leonie that this is typical. The loss of depth perception is profoundly disorienting, and it takes a while for the brain to adjust to monocular vision. But perhaps the more significant hurdle to his recovery is the psychological struggle he may have. Leonie will have to observe for signs that he is failing to cope with the adaptation to his new, altered reality.

Leonie gets to know Hemi well over this period. She admires his attitude, how he remains articulate about the emotions he is experiencing. He is determined to heal, both physically and spiritually. When the time comes, he plans to bury his enucleated eye at his marae.

'How are you feeling?' Leonie asks him.

'I'm OK,' he says. 'Funny, but I feel like I've learned from all this,' he says. 'It has been really enlightening. I've tried to throw all my resources into healing. Having a positive life philosophy and my tikanga Māori has really helped. This hasn't necessarily been a tragedy,' he adds.

Leonie has learned, too, and far more than just some of the techniques of caring for those who have suffered eye trauma. She has learned much about resilience, and about how and where we look within ourselves for healing.

He pō, he pō
He ao, he ao
Tākiri mai te ata
Korihi te manu
Ka ao, ka ao
Ka ao te rā

Darkness, darkness
Light, light
Day has dawned
The birds are singing
It is light, it is light
The sun is shining

This is not the first serious eye injury Leonie has dealt with on the island. Several years earlier, a patient had presented unremarkably to the front desk of the health centre with his fist clamped over his left eye. Leonie ambled over to his side as she passed through the waiting room, and was immediately struck by how pale he was.

'You'd better come with me,' she said, and led him into the nurse's station. 'What happened?'

'I was at home putting a window into my excavator. Slowly, as I fed the rubber weather strip around, I needed to lever it in tighter with one of the two screwdrivers I had. I just needed to put a bit more pressure on . . . then it slipped. *Ping!* Straight in my eye. *Oh hell*, I think. Thirty seconds later I'm thinking, *Well, I can think. That must mean I'm not dead.* Praise God I'm still alive and the screwdriver didn't get to my brain. I knew I needed help, so I put the dogs away in their pen then drove here.'

'You drove yourself?'

'Yes. First gear all the way. What else could I do?' He grinned. 'Not sure how I made it, but here I am.'

Leonie was horrified. She peered to see if she could see the offending screwdriver protruding from his eye. All she could see was his hand. She settled him on the examination couch and dashed off to locate Ivan.

As Leonie organised the intravenous pain relief and anti-emetic, Ivan scrubbed up and peered closely into the left eye.

'You have a disrupted orbit,' Ivan pronounced.

'What's that in English?' the digger driver asked with a grin.

'I can't tell exactly what you've done to the inner structures, but I can see the wound involves your cornea and I can see bits of your iris protruding. There's a large blood clot beyond that, so I can't see what's happening at the back.'

The eye specialists at Auckland Hospital would likely inspect it all under a general anaesthetic, he added.

The patient needed no persuasion to be evacuated immediately to the mainland. Leonie made the arrangements, and then rang around until she located the patient's son.

Minutes later, he was there.

'Dad! What have you done to yourself?' he asked.

His dad explained, and then calmly issued instructions on what needed doing around home. By now, Leonie had dressed his eye, and the pain relief was working well. His vital signs were stable. Soon the helicopter arrived to whisk him off to Auckland Hospital, still in his work clothes and hefty boots.

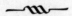

Nor is Hemi the last to lose his vision in Leonie's time, although the third case is not the result of trauma. One day, a local woman—a farmer—presents complaining of a loss of vision in her right eye.

'I just woke up and I went to look at Pitokuku.' She names the hill beside her home, the prospect of which she has always called her favourite view. 'I was just looking like I usually do at the clouds— you know, to see what way the wind's blowing, if there's rain. I always do that. But this morning I couldn't see it properly. I ducked my head under the blankets and popped it out again, but I still couldn't see properly.'

In reply to their questions, she tells Ivan and Leonie that she can see normally out of her left eye, but when she covers that eye and tries to look out of her right . . . darkness. Maybe there are dim shadows, grey patches, but otherwise everything is black.

'So I woke Charlie and told him, "I can't see", and he told me not to be so damn stupid. But maybe he did care, because he disappears and fetches our daughter.'

Their daughter is a trained nurse. She knew this was serious, and sent them to the health centre at once.

'Is there any pain?' Ivan asks.

'No, thankfully not. No pain. I just can't see out of this eye.' Her voice wobbles, and a tear trickles down her face. 'When I try to look out of only my right eye it's like being in the bush at night and trying to look up and see the sky. It's all so dark. It's like trying to look out from a room when all the windows on one side are blanked out . . . That's the only words I have to describe it.'

Leonie is called away again—it's a very busy Saturday morning in January at the health centre—and when she comes back, Ivan has put drops in the woman's eye to dilate the pupil. He is taking a history, and she is answering his questions with good-humoured impatience.

'No, Ivan,' she says. 'There's no history of diabetes in my family. You know that. Everyone in my family's one of your patients.'

'High blood pressure?'

She rolls her eyes—the good one and the one from which she can't see. 'No, Ivan. No high blood pressure.'

Ivan is consulting her notes.

'Yes, Ivan. I turned sixty-six in October. No, I definitely have not taken up smoking.'

Her blood pressure and pulse are normal. Ivan darkens the room and explains the eye examination he is about the perform. She sits still and compliant. Her eye shines like a jewel in the concentrated light of his ophthalmoscope. He leans this way and that, viewing from different angles, and Leonie imagines what this examination would have been like in the caravan.

'OK,' he says, rocking back on his heels. 'I've been looking at the back of your eye. It looks to me like you've got a central retinal vein occlusion, which is a blockage in one of the blood vessels that supplies blood from your retina. I'm not a hundred per cent sure, because there is a pale optic disc back there too, and I don't know why. It's not typical of a vein occlusion.'

'What does all that mean?' the patient asks.

Ivan frowns. 'I'm not sure, until I've talked to the eye specialists at the hospital. Can you remember what you were doing yesterday? Was it stressful?'

She is momentarily at a loss.

'Oh, I remember,' she says. 'We had a stall at the New Year's Picnic. What a carry-on that was. I was flat-out all day, you know, organising everything and then running the stall. Makes me tired just thinking about it. But, oh, yes . . .' She pauses for a moment. 'When we got home, it was dark. I distinctly remember standing outside with my granddaughter and we just looked up at the glorious night sky. The stars were terrific. It seemed like I could see forever. I thought, *How special is that?*'

Ivan phones Auckland Hospital as the patient lies on the couch, trying to make sense of the technical terms she overhears. She begins to cry again, the tears spilling down her face.

The hospital doctors want Ivan to keep her under observation for the rest of the day. He gives her an aspirin, to help with thinning the blood and reducing any clotting. Leonie makes up a bed for her in the 'ward', which is an adjacent room where there are mattresses on the floor at this time of year to cope with the big influx of patients over the period on either side of New Year's. The patient lies there drifting in and out of sleep all day, Leonie or Ivan checking in from time to time, with her family dropping by to visit. Late in the afternoon, she is given a final orbital massage, as prescribed by the hospital, and Ivan performs another full eye examination.

'The hospital can see you on Monday,' Ivan says, after he has phoned the mainland to report his findings.

The patient looks dismayed. 'Don't they want to see me straight away?' she asks.

'No, they feel we can wait,' Ivan replies.

He and Leonie can see the significance dawning upon her. The tears start again. They try to allay her anxiety but she tells them that this is the scariest thing that has ever happened to her.

'You can go home. I would like you to come back tomorrow morning so we can review your eye again. And, in the meantime, Leonie will make you up a dressing that will make you look like a pirate.'

The patient smiles through her tears.

The outcome, as Ivan had feared, was the confirmation of a central retinal occlusion and the complete loss of vision in that eye. There was no reason found for the pale optic disc, though it was of interest to the specialists. It was suggested that the previous day's stress may have contributed to the event. With all the empathy in the world, you cannot really appreciate the impact of a sudden loss of this magnitude unless you have experienced it.

This would have been a terrifying and isolating time for this woman. Word got around about her misfortune, as it does in the island community, and the excavator driver did not hesitate to step forward and offer his wholehearted support. After all, he had walked the same dark path.

On a day when she was feeling her loss particularly, he gave her a neck massage and listened as she poured out her fears and regrets and gently reminded her that her life would go on, and that, with time, she would adjust.

And adjust she has.

'You should see me trying to thread a needle, Leonie!' She laughs. 'And if someone over there—' she gestures off to the right— 'talks to me, I've got to turn my whole body around to look at them. And I'm a shocker for clipping people as I walk past them. They must think I'm awfully rude. I tell them I'm sorry, but I'm glad we don't have big crowds on the Barrier. Imagine me in Auckland! My grandson holds my hand crossing the road.'

She shows Leonie her range of walking sticks. The paddocks on her farm are far from even, and she has to be careful. And when she is mustering she has to constantly turn her head or even turn completely around to make sure her dogs have not left any sheep behind.

'I get dizzy, too,' she says. 'If I move suddenly, everything spins for a minute. The others tell me they get that too. It took me a few falls to get my head around that one.'

'But you are OK?' Leonie asks.

'I'm OK,' she replies. 'I can still work the farm. I can still do my quilting.' She pauses, and a range of emotions cross her face. 'And I can still look at the stars with my granddaughter,' she says.

Chapter 9

PROGRESS

Probably the greatest challenge for the island's health professionals is the sheer relentlessness of being on-call. For the best part of the first fifteen years after we each began, Adele was on-call for those in the isolated north of the island while Leonie and Ivan cared for the bulk of those in the middle and south of the island. With solid support from Nancy (and, after her retirement in 1991, her replacement, Peter) this was of course on top of our full daily clinical load—cradle-to-grave primary healthcare.

While one of the major attractions of life on the Barrier is the outdoors—the bush and the sea—we were unable, for a long time, to make the most of it, as we were obliged to be constantly contactable. You couldn't have a day at the beach without letting someone (usually, at first, one or other of the telephone operators) know exactly where you were. And even at night you were always on-call.

In the period just after the births of Amiria and Jordan, Leonie's children, life was pretty intense. Leonie had to juggle breastfeeding with full-time work and being on-call. It didn't help that the island was experiencing a minor baby boom all of its own, with around 30 pregnancies a year requiring antenatal and postnatal care and, in many cases, midwifery services at the birth (compared with the more usual ten per annum nowadays). The silver lining of the workload that this entailed is that Leonie shared the journey through the infancy of her children with other mothers who (life on Aotea being as it is) were also juggling multiple responsibilities—breastfeeding, home-based businesses, part-time employment and the simple, hard, diligent effort it is to cook, clean and do laundry in the absence of reticulated electricity, and using alternative energy systems like wind, solar and hydro, which are at the mercy of vagaries in the weather.

This group of young mums shared a common bond. Leonie revelled in the support of like-minded women, and she also appreciated several meaningful relationships based on her Christian beliefs. They laughed and cried together, and ultimately were empowered by the experience of sharing some of the special moments in one another's lives.

It is all very well that nurses, like everyone, are encouraged to lead a balanced lifestyle, keeping a proper work–life balance; this all goes out the window in a remote place like Aotea. And island nursing can be difficult enough without having to wear the yoke of perfection. Balancing the roles of 'good nurse', 'good wife' and 'good mother' can be tricky. It is easy enough to put your patients' needs before your own, but it is hard to put them before your children's interests. This is exactly what the job often required Leonie to do, and her bad case of the working mum's guilts became even worse when Ivan was called out alongside her. But on-call work can also be intensely rewarding; some of Leonie's most satisfying nursing moments have come when she and Ivan have been on-call.

When the children were very young, Leonie and Ivan perfected the art of waking them, grabbing their pillows and a blanket, and racing off to the health centre, where Amiria and Jordan quickly learned to snuggle down in a quiet space on the carpet and fall back to sleep. On one memorable occasion, the children were woken by the squall of a newborn baby: a mother had given birth before her due date. Far from being put out, they were excited. This was a break from routine! They loved saying hello to the wee baby.

One night, when her daughter Amiria wasn't quite two, Leonie spied on her through her bedroom doorway and watched, bemused, as she ferreted through a drawer, strewing clothes on the floor, before she seemed to settle on a selection, which she carefully stacked on the end of her bed.

'What are you doing?' Leonie asked.

'These are what I want to wear tomorrow,' Amiria replied in a very grown-up voice.

As Leonie tucked her into bed, she suddenly realised what was going on. She, too, was in the habit of placing a stack of clothes at the end of the bed, just in case she was called out in the wee hours. Amiria was simply following suit.

Years later, when Jordan skipped home from school one Friday, he looked at Ivan and said, 'Are we on-call this weekend?'

When Jordan was around three, a local woman named Cherie approached Leonie and Ivan and told them how much she enjoyed Jordan's company. 'Would you like some support?' she wondered. 'Would it be OK if Jordan—and perhaps Amiria too—spent time with my family?

Would it ever!

Cherie became the Howie children's 'other mother'. It has proved to be a great relationship for both families. Both Amiria and Jordan relished the opportunities that being part of Cherie's family provided, and being able to make the absolute most of the outdoor heaven that the Barrier provides—surfing, swimming, fishing, biking, trail-biking, going rabbiting. Cherie thought herself lucky that the children enjoyed all the things she loved doing. Cherie played a large part in providing Jordan and Amiria with an idyllic childhood—so much so that their big brother, Alastair, would comment how lucky they were. He spent every school holiday that he possibly could on the island, but by now he was at university. He loved the island and would disappear for hours mountain-biking, swimming or just walking, revelling in being a Barrierite again whenever he returned. These days, when the two younger Howie children return to the island, Cherie's home is one of their first ports of call.

Many was the time that Ivan and Leonie found themselves unable to take the children with them on a call-out. At such times, they were always able to fling Jordan and Amiria at Cherie and her family, no matter what time of the day or night.

The children were, as children are, very adaptable. They didn't seem to mind sharing their parents with the community. They learned to be creative with their time. Once, when they were in their twenties, Leonie asked them whether they minded growing up as part of the Howie Health Team.

Both merely shrugged. 'It's all we knew. No problems, Mum,' they answered.

Leonie let out a sigh of relief. Both had normalised their growing-up experiences.

And, in fact, they occasionally remind Leonie of the little ways in which they have been useful to the health team.

'Remember when the Health Trust bought the new ear microscope, Mum, and we became the guinea pigs?' Jordan says. 'You and Dad had us up on the table practising looking down it.'

'Actually,' chimes in Amiria, 'I remember when the man was demonstrating to Dad the finer points of the ultrasound machine. I ended up with all the ultrasound gel on my stomach.'

'Did we do that?' Leonie says. 'How awful! I am sure that must be unethical—doing medical experiments on your own children.'

'Oh, that wasn't so bad. The worst was when Dad decided to burn off my warts with the frecator when he was showing the other GP how to use it.'

—⋙—

The islanders understood perfectly well what being on-call meant for us, and both of us can remember occasions where we knew for certain that people had put off seeking medical attention just so that we were not called out after-hours.

Leonie remembers one Monday morning, for example, when an elderly gentleman presented himself to the clinic as the very first patient—in considerable pain.

'What have you done to yourself?' Leonie asked.

'My daft draft horse has trodden on my big toe,' he replied. 'Hurt a bit, I can tell you.'

'When did this happen?' Leonie asks.

'Saturday morning,' he replies.

Predictably, the toe is crushed and beyond repair. Ivan explains that it will need to be amputated.

'Why didn't you call us sooner?' Leonie asked.

'Oh.' He smiled serenely. 'Well, the toe wasn't going anywhere fast.'

Leonie was blessed to have a number of close, loving friends from the mainland who became an anchor during stressful times. They would arrive laden with treats—'Red Cross parcels'—from across the Hauraki Gulf and save the day. And Leonie's mum, Isabel, herself a rural nurse earlier in life, would visit for four to six weeks over the busy summer season, when the huge visiting population meant everything would become frantic and Leonie's workload would more than double.

Isabel was the matriarch of the Taylors until she died in her early nineties. She had not only cared for her own extended family in Northland, but she had for a time also worked in the local maternity hospital to supplement the income from the family farm. She understood Leonie's nursing values, as they replicated her own. She understood implicitly whenever Leonie disappeared to 'nurse'. Her summer visits to the Barrier were often to her own, personal cost—either her cat would disappear, or her neglected garden would shrivel up under the blazing Northland sun. She would miss out on wider family gatherings at the bach and fail to connect with her childhood friends who returned to their families for the holiday season but would be gone when she returned in February.

Essentially, she would run the Howie household, caring for the children, preparing the meals and entertaining any visitors. She never neglected her post, even when invited out by a persistent, on-island suitor she had somehow acquired. Amiria and Jordan adored her. When Aotea Health had reached the point where it was no longer an inexcusable extravagance to hire a locum, Leonie, Ivan and the children would holiday up at her home on the family farm at least once a year.

Adele spent much of this period of her life in the north of the island juggling responsibilities, too. Soon after she and Shannon started their mussel-farming venture, they commissioned the building of a seeding and harvesting barge in cooperation with two of the other new mussel-farm owners. Around the same time, Adele entered the joint venture with Ivan and Leonie in the formation of Aotea Health Limited. She found herself running the books for the mussel-farm ventures and for Aotea Health, as well as working full-time as a rural nurse and midwife.

Mussel harvesting often took place on the weekend, and Adele came to dread early-morning phone calls, as these days it was less likely to be a woman in labour than someone phoning to say they could not come to work on the barge that day. On such mornings, Shannon would ask her to get out of bed and come and help on the marine farm.

'No! No! I already have a job!' she would groan.

Once she got out there in the still of the bay, with birdsong floating across the water from the bush, Adele usually found herself enjoying the work, along with the repartee among the crew—to say nothing of the steamed-mussel sandwiches they had for lunch.

But being in charge of the books exposed Adele to the grinding anxiety that is making a living in primary production. She and Shannon once had the unenviable experience of watching, sick at heart, as the news on national television carried pictures of 40 tonnes of their mussels being dumped in a Tauranga landfill due to a toxic algal bloom. Or she would note the rise in the Kiwi dollar against New Zealand's export partners and see a season's hard work and a bumper crop realise next to nothing. Or the exchange rate and the market price would both be favourable, but for some reason or another— poor seed uptake, snapper attack on juvenile seed, overgrowth of black mussels—they would have a meagre harvest.

Often Adele found herself crying as she drove home in the dark at the end of a long, stressful day. It was like her first six months on the island all over again.

By now, she and Shannon had shifted out of the nurse's cottage and were living in their own very small house. The telephone was in the lounge so that it was easily accessible when Adele was on-call, and Shannon began complaining that, because she was always on the phone, he couldn't make the calls he needed to for the mussel-farming venture. One day, frustrated, Adele phoned Telecom and asked for another line to be installed to the house. It quickly became apparent that the phone rang for him just as often as it rang for her.

'Your phone's ringing,' she would say with a smile as yet another dinner or TV show was interrupted.

The busy—at times, frantic—life we lead often makes us think about the lives of those who had preceded us on Aotea. Adele has been something of a collector of stories and anecdotes of the old-time nurses on the island: locals and visitors have given her snippets of information, and her own research has filled in some of the gaps. Looking at their lives makes us realise that hardship has always been part of the fabric of nursing on the island, although less so as time passes.

One of the earliest reports of a nurse on Great Barrier Island was Elizabeth Medland (née Stringer), who married Thomas Medland, one of the original farmers on the island. She arrived as a young bride in the 1870s. She was a Salvationist whose vocation it was to provide help to any who required it. The first nurse to be officially appointed to the island as a midwife was Annie Medland, Elizabeth's daughter, who left the island specifically to train so that she could return and serve the community. She was to be the second of four generations of nurses in her family. Annie was registered as a midwife in 1923. She returned home during the First World War and worked on a voluntary basis until 1929, when we believe she was appointed to the position by the Auckland Hospital Board.

In 1927, Judy McLean moved to the island to farm with her husband. She had trained at Gisborne and Taihape Hospitals. Their farm was in Nagle Cove, an isolated bay in the northern part of the island with no road access. Just like Annie Medland, Judy worked on a voluntary basis, responding to neighbours and other islanders when called upon. In 1933, she was appointed district nurse by the Auckland Hospital Board, a position she held until 1944 when she and her husband sold the farm and moved off the island. In 1947, she was invested with an MBE for her services to Aotea. Her story is all the more remarkable for the fact that she was married; in that era, women did not usually work after marriage. Indeed, Adele once visited an elderly widower who told her that his wife had trained as a nurse before they came to live on the island.

'Did she work as a nurse?' Adele asked.

'No, definitely not!' the man replied, shocked. 'She was married!'

Some still remember Judy McLean. They remember her arriving on her horse, beautifully dressed in her riding gear, with polished boots and saddlebags. Her regular monthly trips lasted a week, as she would stay at various homesteads along the way—longer if she arrived at a home where the mother was ill, because she thought nothing of staying a few days to assist with the running of the house.

Mrs McLean and the early nurses rode to Katherine Bay (one of the last places on the island to get a driveable road) every fortnight—a trip that now takes Adele 25 minutes, but used to take Judy two hours over a very steep and rough bridle track. Judy's daughter said that she once asked her mother why she was so grumpy when she arrived home from these trips. The next time she went, Judy took her daughter with her on the extremely long and tiring day. They were both grumpy at the end of it.

In 1937, during Judy's tenure, there was an outbreak of typhoid fever among the Māori community at Katherine Bay. Mrs McLean stayed with them for a week, helping to nurse those affected and to educate people about typhoid and how to avoid contracting it; the community had thought that the sickness had come about because of a curse. The Department of Health flew in to investigate and to immunise 87 people in the four affected settlements. A newspaper article at the time made much of the heroic exploits of the Medical Officers of Health but made no mention of the resident nurse.

In 1946, Edna Metcalfe—known to all and sundry as Ted—was the first nurse to be appointed public health nurse to Aotea who did not have a personal connection with the island. She had travelled and nursed extensively overseas before her stint on Great Barrier Island, and she did more travelling afterwards. She and five subsequent nurses were accommodated at Glenfern—also called FitzRoy House—at Port FitzRoy, across the bay from the wharf. Their daily commute involved rowing across the bay to the wharf, or riding up and around the head of the bay on horseback. During Ted's time, the nurses were supplied with a 1939 Chevrolet, but the roads were such that not all areas were accessible by car. Katherine Bay was still only accessible on horseback. After Mrs McLean, the horses used belonged to the Coopers at Okiwi, of whom Garth Cooper, the Okiwi telephone exchange operator, was one. A vehicular road finally reached Katherine Bay in 1956.

The fifth public health nurse on Aotea, Muriel, started in 1948.

She was given a farewell by the community at Port FitzRoy the following year—only to return a short time later married to Laurie Curreen, who farmed at Awana. The locals thought this was both hilarious and mystifying: on an island where everyone more or less knows everyone else's business, they had not seen that one coming at all. There had been speculation, but in another direction completely. Adele actually knew Muriel, and attended when, in her eighties, she passed away in the presence of her daughter (also a nurse) and son, at home. Driving through the Awana valley, she still finds herself looking for Muriel in her wide-brimmed hat with a basket, collecting wild mushrooms from the farm paddocks.

Phyllis Wharfe, the ninth nurse, held the position on the island from 1953 until 1958. Although Miss Wharfe had a car, the roads were unsealed and there were still twenty gates to open on her journey the length of the island. She made regular, three-month visits aboard a naval vessel, HMNZFA *Endeavour*, to the lighthouse families on the Cuvier and Mokohinau islands. Miss Wharfe was held in very high regard by the people of Great Barrier Island, and the feeling was mutual: she told a newspaper that 'the people on the island are extremely hospitable and cooperative, and in cases of serious sickness or accidents will do everything possible to assist the nurse. Their launches, rowing boats and horses are at the nurse's disposal at any time the need arises.'

Phyllis Wharfe took a keen interest in the dream of young Grace Benson (née Medland), who was inspired by her family's involvement in nursing on the island and also by her admiration for Mrs McLean and Miss Wharfe. In 1954, Miss Wharfe took Grace along when she walked to Whangaparapara from Claris (there was a slip on the road) to visit a family living near the whaling station. When Grace left the island in 1956 to train as a nurse, Phyllis kept in touch with her, and in 1959 sent her a white handkerchief to mark her graduation.

The nurse's cottage was built between the wharf and the shop at Port FitzRoy in 1956 by Harry and his brother Chris Ngawaka, and it is still in operation today. In 1989, when an upgrade of the septic tank system was contemplated, Adele received a phone call from her superiors in Auckland asking her whether it was possible that the Auckland Hospital Board did not own the land where the house was situated. The best information they had been able to find seemed to suggest that it had belonged to the Forest Service, and was therefore now owned by the Department of Conservation.

Adele laughed. 'It's totally possible,' she said. 'They were simpler times. Government departments talked to each other in those days, and they actually cooperated. I can imagine the Department of Health talking to the Forest Service and saying, "We need to build a clinic for the Great Barrier Island nurses", and both agreeing on a suitable site. It would have just been "government land".'

That struck her as typical of Great Barrier Island. So, too, did the fact that, when the nurse's cottage was upgraded after the Community Trust took over ownership in 1994, it was Harry's son Opo and Harry and Chris's nephew Aaron who performed the work.

There was a high turnover of nurses once Phyllis Wharfe left. Some are remembered kindly; others less so. There are many stories. Adele was told of a close predecessor of hers, a colourful nurse who also had her pilot's licence. None of the locals were game to fly with her because she also rode a motorbike.

'If she flies like she rides,' they would say, 'no way am I getting in an aeroplane with her!'

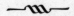

In 1991, Nancy retired. This was a wrench: she was such a support for both of us in our early days, and even now we regard her as a mentor. But she was replaced as part-time public health nurse based in Tryphena, at the southern end of the island, by Peter, who transferred from the public sector to become Aotea Health's first bona-fide employee in 1994. He joked that he thought being in management was a bigger risk than being an employee, so he chose to become an employee. He has been a stalwart of our health team ever since. His official title is rural nurse specialist, and his role encompasses community mental health and emergency specialities along with the usual range of regular health-centre clinical work that we all perform.

When he is not nursing, Peter farms a 115-acre property at Taylors Bay on the southern side of the entrance to Tryphena Harbour—the scene, incidentally, of one of the Barrier's more notorious claims to fame due to a murder that happened there in 1886. A settler known as 'Tusky' Taylor farmed there and was killed by a man who arrived with the avowed intention of abducting his daughter, Elizabeth. Elizabeth evaded him, and the murderer and an accomplice were eventually caught in Sydney, then tried and executed in Auckland.

When Peter first arrived, the wild cattle that frequently emerged from the bush and crossed his land kept his family in meat. Nowadays he has orchards and his own livestock that he farms over his predominantly bush-clad land. Peter is a gifted storyteller and enjoys regaling us with snippets from his life. From his pig-story repertoire, the most memorable ones describe his relationship with 'Feral Cheryl'.

Peter first met Feral Cheryl when he and his partner, Wendy, were driving home from the health centre in Claris one Christmas Eve. As they were driving up Medland Road, he rounded a corner and spied a small wild piglet foraging at the roadside. He braked hard and pulled off the road.

'I'm going to catch that pig,' he told Wendy.

He jumped out of the car and, as the piglet ran off, he gave chase, staying on the seaward side of the road. To his right the road fell away into dense scrub, and that is where the piglet wanted to be. The road on its left-hand side cut into the hillside, and so the piglet was forced to run along the bank with Peter pelting along beside it.

He saw the moment at which the piglet decided it was not going to outrun him. Instead, it tried scrambling up the steep bank, but quickly realised this was futile. So instead, it rounded on Peter, growling and snapping. Peter grabbed the piglet and carried it, squealing and wriggling, back to his car. Wendy was none too keen on it—and less keen when she found it was covered in lice—but Peter soon won both Wendy and Feral Cheryl (as he named her) over to the idea of having (and being) a pet pig. Over the next three years, he kept us entertained with stories of Feral Cheryl's exploits. We even have a photograph on the team noticeboard from the early days that showed him fast asleep in a favourite chair, with a tiny piglet on his lap, also fast asleep, with its wee snout in the air.

Later in life, of course, Feral Cheryl grew to be a gigantic sow with a capacity for eating everything and anything.

The next addition to Aotea Health's payroll was Peter's partner, Wendy, our part-time receptionist at the community health centre in the middle of the island. Wendy was a retired psychiatric nurse with an excellent grasp of office management, an understanding of medical confidentiality and amazing people skills. She fitted the role perfectly. Over time, our administrative and support staff has increased, but Leonie remembers just how luxurious it seemed to finally have someone else to act as the first point of contact with our patients, even if it was only for a few hours a week.

Of course, by 1997, the real need was for an additional general practitioner. Ivan had by now been working as the island's sole GP for nearly sixteen years, on-call 24 hours and seven days a week. We often talked about how good it would be to recruit another doctor— especially if that doctor were a woman, so that we could offer a choice to the islanders. But we had no accommodation to offer, and the finances would only allow for a very small part-time position.

Ivan and Leonie have a deep Christian faith and proposed that they would pray for a doctor to be sent to the island. After waiting some time, Adele suggested that we might have to be a bit more proactive and advertise. The Howies had planned a holiday, so it was decided to defer the discussion until their return. It is fair to say, though, that Adele wasn't holding her breath.

Then one day, shortly after they had left and Adele was looking after the reception while the receptionist was off at lunch, a woman walked in.

'Hello,' Adele said. 'Can I help you?'

'Hi,' the woman answered in an English accent. 'I'm a doctor—a general practitioner—and I've just moved to the island. I was wondering if you would have any work for me. I can only work one or two days a week, but, well, I thought I would ask . . .You know, on the off-chance.'

Adele realised she was staring, open-mouthed.

She couldn't wait for Leonie and Ivan to get back to give them this amazing piece of news. Sarah subsequently worked with us, part-time, for five years.

For the islanders, one of the changes we have been able to make since the health reforms and the creation of Aotea Health is being able to place a rural lens over all our contracts and any policies that come our way. Using the islanders' experience, we have become skilled at identifying and hopefully rectifying potential pitfalls. Through this lobbying, our team now includes two full-time general practitioner positions. Previously, there was little chance we could have attracted doctors to the island, because it would take a special sort of person to accept the crushing on-call load that the sole-charge GP shouldered: so far as we could tell, Ivan was one of a kind. Similarly, while we knew we had become adept at wearing many hats as nurses on Aotea, we were quite chuffed to see how many scopes of nursing practice our contracts covered: a 'rural nurse' on Aotea is a practice nurse, a district nurse, a public health nurse, a palliative care nurse, a child health nurse and a school nurse. Creating Aotea Health has enabled us to share the load with other nursing members, who work on a part-time basis but still carry an on-call load. And of course, all good health teams rely heavily on administration staff and Aotea Health is no different: we have been lucky in our loyal team members. Not that we have been able to put our feet up! The two of us remain full-time rural nurse specialists and rural midwives, in addition to our management load.

We all belong, all of us part of the community in which we work. For some, personal career changes and shifting family needs have necessitated moves back to the mainland. These nurses and doctors remain in touch, still interested in the island and its people. There is something about Aotea and what you are part of when you work here—involved in the islanders' lives from cradle to grave—that leaves its mark.

The Great Barrier Island Community Health Trust has stood beside us all the way, providing the nuts and bolts to keep our service running with well-maintained buildings and vehicles for us to lease. Expensive medical equipment materialises from tireless fundraising and ensures that we no longer feel we are attending emergencies with a Band-Aid.

We have also come a long way since Adele was first responder to the car off the road at Kōtuku Peninsula. Emergency care services on the island have evolved, too. The Ministry of Health and ACC commenced a scheme known as PRIME (Primary Response In Medical Emergencies) to facilitate improved pre-hospital emergency care in rural New Zealand. Successive island doctors and nurses have received specialised emergency training. And whereas the New Zealand Police—most of the time, the sole-charge Great Barrier Island policeman—used to provide the ambulance service, for the last five years St John have joined the island's emergency team, operating as a First Response Unit and providing ambulance support. An experienced St John manager came to live on Aotea and offered to set up a service to complement the health team. He himself has retrained to paramedic level and is extremely competent, and, following his lead, some of the locals have volunteered and become skilled practitioners too, moving up through the ranks. It is encouraging to see the long hours of training they invest in helping their fellow community members. This collaborative emergency team approach can also involve the police, the Great Barrier Voluntary Fire Force, the Coastguard and the Civil Defence team. All have been staunch in their ongoing support, dealing with emergencies together in the time-honoured Barrier way—part and parcel of island life.

All the same, and with all the latest and best procedures, personnel and protocols in place, the Barrier sometimes has a way of making events dance to the beat of its own, unique drum.

It is the Christmas holidays, and Jill's two older sons are over on the island, as they usually are at this time of the year. Jill tells Leonie that they love making the most of everything the Barrier and their bay has to offer. This year the eldest has brought his pregnant wife.

'Oh?' Leonie's ears prick up. 'How pregnant?'

It turns out she is only a little over 26 weeks along, but Leonie does not relax. She knows from experience that, the moment you take such things for granted, they have a habit of setting you straight. She often hears people—locals and visitors alike—sigh, 'Oh, everything will be fine. It is only the early days of the pregnancy and there are midwives on the island.' Their blind faith in our services has a habit of backfiring when an emergency arises and it is the middle of a foul night when aircraft are grounded.

One January day, Jill's daughter-in-law presents to Leonie, who is on her own midwifery-wise; Ivan and Adele are both away in the north seeing patients. Jill has noted the young woman's headache and puffy feet and hands and has correctly decided these are worrying enough symptoms this early in the pregnancy to encourage her to check things out with Leonie. The mum-to-be is not overly worried herself; she is only just over 26 weeks, but would prefer to have some reassurance. She chattily tells Leonie that she dropped into the cafe on the way and picked up a slice of their amazing sticky date cake to enjoy later as she reads a few magazines.

Leonie is only half listening, because she is looking at the blood pressure reading and becoming alarmed. It is high, and throughout the visit, each time she measures it again, it is rising—dangerously so. Nor is the swelling limited to a bit of puffiness about her hands and feet: the skin of her calves and wrists is stretched taut. The conclusive test is the urine. There is protein present, and these three signs, together with the history of headache are indicative of an escalating emergency—a fulminating (rapidly deteriorating) pre-eclampsia.

Leonie explains her suspicions to the young woman.

'I was only reading about that the other day,' she says, horrified.

'I won't start fitting, will I? Will this harm our baby?'

Leonie offers what reassurance she can and suggests arranging an emergency evacuation to the mainland and specialist care at National Women's Hospital. The patient, shocked at this rapidly escalating scenario, offers no resistance, and Leonie phones an obstetrician to devise a care plan. The helicopter is summoned.

While they are waiting, the young woman is preoccupied with trying to alert her husband. Leonie has already asked Jill to find him, but Jill tells her that, confident all was well with his wife, he has left on a diving trip with her own partner. Leonie sits with her patient, breathing slowly and calmly and encouraging her to do the same, but leaves the room every now and then to try Jill again. It is all she can do to keep herself from yelling down the phone, 'What? You still haven't found him?'

'There's no marine radio on the boat,' Jill says. 'I'm doing everything I can.'

Leonie pauses before returning to the room where the patient is lying, and takes a deep breath to restore her aura of serenity. This takes some doing, as the moment is fast approaching where she will have to despatch this concerned young woman alone on the Auckland Rescue Helicopter. If her husband is not on that flight, it will be a long time before he catches up with her.

To make matters worse, Leonie has other patients. It is high summer—peak season at the health centre—and she has to balance her nursing duties with this emergency.

The phone rings with the news that the helicopter has been delayed. Jill's daughter-in-law is keeping it together, but the anxiety is not helping her hypertension. Just before the aircraft's revised time of arrival, a young man strides into the health centre dressed in a wetsuit, a swipe of sunblock across his nose, ghostly pale and still clutching his catch bag (with live crayfish scratching about inside it).

'You made it,' Leonie says.

Jill's son nods, even as the windows begin vibrating with the beat of the rotors. A short time later, the helicopter paramedic arrives, accompanied by a cameraman who is shooting a reality-TV show. There is no time to waste, and the patient, her husband and his crays are all loaded aboard and the helicopter lifts off without delay.

Leonie later learns the details of how Jill alerted her son to his wife's plight. Jill, at her wits' end, decided to telephone the local marine radio channel. They obligingly put a call out over channel sixteen, the emergency frequency, detailing the boat, the men aboard and the need for their urgent return. The locals knew Jill's partner's boat well, but there was still no response. George, the radio operator, decided to call in favours. He knew the RNZAF Orion was involved in an exercise nearby, so he alerted them to join the search.

The men had just surfaced after a successful cray dive. As they were waiting on the surface, the Orion scribed a circle low above them, then another, each time dipping its wing.

'Jill wants you to hurry home!' one of the men joked, and they both laughed. But the Orion came back and performed another double circuit, dipping its wing, and their smiles disappeared. Something serious was afoot.

Once aboard, the boat sped to the wharf at Whangaparapara, just around from Okupu, where someone shouted to them that both Jill and her daughter-in-law had been involved in a car accident. They were seriously injured and were about to be air-lifted to Auckland Hospital.

We often find that stories are muddled in times of emergency as they are passed between people.

Jill's partner gave his engines all they had on the trip around to

Okupu. He was relieved to see Jill standing at the head of the bay waving them in. Their relief was short-lived. When the correct details were relayed, her son jumped back in the boat, was ferried at speed to the wharf from where a car whisked him to the health centre, just in time to be evacuated with his wife.

The pre-eclampsia was managed by the specialists at National Women's, and in the fullness of time Jill's daughter-in-law delivered Jill her first granddaughter. In celebration of the birth, Jill gave Leonie a handcrafted wooden trug, which takes pride of place on top of her fridge and which she loads with flowers and vegetables in season. It is a reminder—as if she is ever likely to forget.

Chapter 10

NO MAN (OR WOMAN) IS AN ISLAND

There are two obvious consequences of living in a place as remote as Great Barrier Island. The first is that it throws people back on the resources available to them—both their own and the community's. The islanders have always been resilient individuals, first as a matter of necessity, and also as a matter of pride. Whereas you may find hospital emergency department waiting rooms filled with people with coughs and colds and non-specific aches and pains, it is unusual to have an islander present with anything trivial. Sometimes, we wish they had a slightly lower threshold.

The other consequence of isolation is that it makes our clinical judgement absolutely critical. We must tread a fine line between being precautionary—if we make the wrong call and fail to send someone off-island for further assessment, it could have profound consequences—or likewise put the islanders to the considerable expense and inconvenience if evacuation to the mainland proves unnecessary.

Of course, things have improved vastly over the thirty years we have practised on the island. In the days when there were no health facilities on the island, people were on their own and so became resourceful. The pioneering and Māori families all have stories of instances of having to deal with emergencies with no available health professionals close by at all. One day, an elderly woman proudly stuck out her arm as Adele was examining her.

'Well, what do you think of that?' she asked.

'Looks like a pretty normal arm to me,' Adele replied.

'Ha!' the woman said. 'I fell out of a tree when I was five years old and it went snap and it was all crooked. My mother pulled it back into alignment and tied a piece of mānuka to it and we all sat back and waited for it to get better.'

The woman pointed at her elderly brother.

'Look at his nose. See anything?'

Adele shook her head.

'Well, he was cut right here,' she indicated the bridge of her nose. 'Talk about bleed! Our mother glued it up with some gum from a tree and it's good as gold. No scar, at all!'

Even today, there is use of rongoā (traditional medicine)—such things as koromiko (a hebe) for digestive health, kawakawa infusions with multiple therapeutic uses. There is also widespread use of mānuka oil and balm that is produced locally on the island.

One of the areas of our practice in which clinical judgement is absolutely critical is in the birthing of babies. As we have mentioned, there is an unstated expectation these days that mothers will have their babies on the island unless there is a good reason why they should not. There are, of course, precedents for this, too. A midwife from the settler families, Ida Gray (née Hight), had birthed three of the seven children she had on her own. Like her twin sister, Muriel, (who went on to marry a Medland), Ida had undergone some nursing training, and she was registered as a midwife in 1926 after training at St Helen's Maternity Hospital. Her first child was stillborn. Her second, third and sixth were managed by others, but she delivered the fourth by herself on the mainland because the doctor who was expected to attend could not make it. Similarly, she managed the fifth and seventh on Aotea herself because Annie Medland, who was the midwife, didn't make it in time. That last child was born at the height of the typhoid outbreak in 1937. According to Ida's daughter, Ida suspected her seventh baby, who died at eight months, was also a victim of the disease—although this was never able to be confirmed.

With her training and all that experience, Ida was granted a midwifery contract by the Auckland Hospital Board in 1938, on a salary of £2 for midwifery work and 15 shillings for travelling expenses.

Adele can only marvel at the strength and courage of Ida and other women like her. She finds inspiration in their stories, even as her own stories unfold.

Adele examines Jenny. She is getting near term in her third pregnancy. She has expressed a determination to have the baby on the island, but Adele is anxious. All the signs are that the baby is going to be very large, which could lead to complications. Adele—and Ivan concurs when she consults him—that Jenny go to the mainland for an ultrasound scan.

When she arrives back on the island, Adele is reassured.

'So we got it wrong?' she asks. 'The baby's not so big after all?'

'No, you were dead right. It's a whopper. They estimate it will be ten pounds.' Jenny smiles. 'They wanted me to stay and have an early induction.'

'So what on earth are you doing back here?' Adele asks, alarmed.

'Relax, Adele. It'll be all right. I just have big babies.'

Over the next couple of weeks, each time Adele and Ivan see each other, they worry about how much more Jenny's baby will have grown. By now, Adele is practising stuck-shoulder manoeuvres in her sleep. But when finally the day of the birth arrives, Jenny gives a few pushes and delivers a ten-and-a-half-pound baby with minimal fuss.

'Well, Jenny!' Adele says. 'You made that look easy! It could have been even bigger and we still would have been OK.'

Jenny smiles. 'Told you so,' she says. 'I wasn't worried. I just have big babies.'

This is Adele's fifth home birth, and it is one where she starts to learn to trust in and listen to the women. Unless there are clear signs to say otherwise, the mother generally knows what will be best for her baby's birth.

Still, there have been many occasions when Adele has been acutely aware of that line between safety and precaution. Early one summer evening, she gets a call from Sarah, three days before her due date.

'Hi, Adele,' Sarah says. 'I hope you don't have anything on today. I have strong contractions and a small show.'

'Have your waters broken and is the baby active?' Adele enquires.

'No and yes,' answers Sarah. 'And, by the way, I've also rung

Emily* to tell her to keep her legs together as I'm going to be needing the midwives!'

Adele laughs. Emily, Sarah's friend, is ten days past her due date.

Sarah and Adele talk frequently over the course of the afternoon as the labour strengthens. Sarah is the second generation to live in her house. Like many of the island women, she has a strong spiritual connection with the land and, more specifically, with the valley that is her home. She is naturally keen for the baby, the first of the third generation, to be born there.

'I woke this morning with the feeling that something special was going to happen,' she tells Adele after she arrives in the evening. 'I slipped into the vege garden early to enjoy the magic of the dawning day. I took Nyal a coffee at seven-thirty and told him he would be having the day off. I knew I was going into labour.'

He grins. 'I told her I'd better get the final coat of paint on the nursery!'

'So we spent the day pottering around the house, finishing off all our chores. I stopped every now and then to let a contraction pass. When there was no doubt about it, I phoned you at midday.'

Adele is listening to the baby's heartbeat, and finds it is very rapid.

'I don't think it's safe to proceed with the birth at home,' she tells Sarah. 'I think we will have to send you over to hospital by helicopter.'

Sarah looks devastated.

'I'll get a second opinion,' Adele says. 'But I want you to be prepared.'

Sarah nods. She later told Adele that she had made an internal commitment to trust her judgement and not to protest if the call was made to go to leave the island.

---

* Not her real name.

Adele phones Aotea Health's other GP, who in turn phones an obstetrician who is experienced in and supportive of home births. He offers a ray of hope.

'Have you been in the bath at all?' Adele asks.

'Yes,' Sarah replies. 'I was in and out of it all afternoon after the contractions started.'

'How hot did you have it?'

'I don't know. Pretty hot. The heat seemed to help.'

Adele reproaches herself for not instructing her to keep the water temperature at or below 38 degrees celsius.

'The doctor says that sometimes the baby's heart rate is high if the mother has been in hot water and that it usually settles,' Adele explains. 'My feeling is that it has been too fast for too long.'

Adele performs another examination. Sarah's temperature is normal, her pulse is normal and her waters have not yet broken. At five centimetres, she is around halfway dilated. But still the foetal heart rate is high. Adele thinks it best to proceed on the assumption that Sarah will be evacuated. Nyal begins packing a bag for them both.

'Who do you think we should get to look after the chooks and feed the cats?' he asks.

As Sarah is pondering this question, Adele is listening to the baby's heartbeat.

'Great! We're back in the normal range,' she says. 'It could be it has settled down.'

There is an anxious wait, but the baby's heart rate stays in the normal range, and they all relax. After two hours of powerful contractions, Sarah's cervix is still at five centimetres, and Adele decides to break the waters to try to bring on the birth.

A backup midwife, has arrived by now. She and Adele examine

the amniotic fluid and note meconium in it—this is a foetal bowel motion, and a reliable indicator that the baby has been under stress in the womb.

'It's thin and brown,' Adele observes. 'Pretty recent, I'd say. Probably only means the baby was in heat distress. Do you agree?'

The midwife nods.

'OK, well we can probably go ahead with the birth here. But we had best get the GP here at the end.'

They phone the GP and ask her to be on hand in case the baby has inhaled any of the amniotic fluid, which can cause a dangerous lung problem, and just in case there is some reason other than heat for the signs of foetal distress and a resuscitation should become necessary.

By now, it has been a long labour. Sarah has endured twelve hours of strong contractions without pain relief. While the breaking of the waters has sped things up, it is still another hour and a half before Adele decides the birth is imminent and summons the GP.

Soon enough, with Nyal encouraging and holding her, Sarah begins a marathon of pushing and finally the baby crowns. As soon as the head is born, the GP suctions the mouth and nose and Adele checks that the cord is not around the baby's neck. Everything seems normal. With the very next contraction, Arwyn Alice, a wet, wrinkled little bundle, slips into the world. Colour and muscle tone are not brilliant—she is a little pale and floppy—but shortly she screws up her face and cries. Adele dries her quickly and gives her to Sarah to hold.

'Such a big head!' Nyal is saying through his tears. 'I thought the head would just keep on coming and coming!'

Arwyn's heartbeat is over 100 beats per minute—quite normal—and once the cord has stopped pulsing, a proud father cuts it. Adele remarks that it is quite a short cord, and observes that research has shown that it starts out the same length in all pregnancies, but gets stretched by the movements of the baby in utero. Girls move less and tend to have shorter cords.

The baby's father has a swift look, and his face is a picture of delight. 'It's a girl,' he tells Sarah. 'Just like we wanted. It's a girl.'

Sarah is nodding.

'A little girl. That figures. Her movements were really gentle in my tummy.'

All proceeds normally after that, and after a few stitches to Sarah's perineum and a vitamin K injection for baby Arwyn to assist with blood clotting, the health team leave the family to bask in the glow of a happy outcome.

'I was that close to sending her over to Auckland,' Adele says as they leave. 'That close.'

One of Adele's earliest supports when she moved to the island was the family who owned the shop. There were three generations living on the island: a grandmother, her daughter and her granddaughter. And now a great granddaughter is on the way.

Trouble is, it is to be Serena's first birth. This is at a time when Adele is not keen on first births on the island, because there is no track record on which to judge how the mother will bear up. Furthermore, it is more common in first pregnancies for the baby to present in a difficult position, which can prolong the labour and wear out both the mother and her supporters—which makes the pain more intense—and also poses the risk of major complications arising. At least if a woman has given birth previously, you know that, all things being equal, she can fit a baby through the birth canal.

So Adele has been encouraging Serena to have her baby on the mainland. But, when she is performing an examination just before Serena is due to leave, she learns that she will be quite alone in the Greenlane Hospital Nurse's Home awaiting the birth: her partner has just started a new job and simply cannot afford to accompany her, given the whole birth and recovery might take two to four weeks. By now, what is more, Adele has become convinced of the rightness of giving birth in surroundings where you are comfortable and in the presence of people whom you choose.

This is ridiculous, she thinks, so she asks Serena's mother and grandmother what their births have been like.

Both shrug. 'No problems at all,' they say.

Adele suggests to Serena that she talk through with her partner, mother and grandparents the possibility of staying and birthing on the island. All are excited at this prospect, so a plan is made. They will use the nurse's cottage—Serena and her partner live in a shed on the property next door to Adele. It has no running hot water, electricity or heating.

So in the early hours of the very next morning, there is a knock at Adele's door and the young couple are standing there with big smiles to say that labour has started.

As with many first births, it is a long and arduous labour. But Serena copes remarkably well—so well, in fact, that late in the afternoon, after she has birthed her daughter in the presence of her partner, Adele and Ivan (who has come to assist), Adele decides it is worth considering first births on the island in future, if the women are certain that they want to do so.

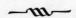

The birth of her daughter is not the last occasion on which Adele witnesses Serena's typical island stoicism and resilience. Around two years after that birth, Adele is sitting writing up her notes. A woman off a boat presented a little earlier with a medical emergency and has just been helicoptered off. Adele happens to glance out the window in time to see Serena walking up to the clinic. As she watches, she notices that Serena is doubled over in obvious pain.

Having seen first-hand how staunch this young woman is and how high her pain threshold, Adele knows this must be something serious. She helps Serena into the clinic and examines her. Serena's description of her symptoms—sudden onset of increasing pain in her pelvic region, a few spots of blood—together with the fact that she has missed two of her periods convinces Adele that they are dealing with an ectopic pregnancy (a potentially life-threatening condition, where a fertilised egg implants somewhere other than in the womb, usually in a fallopian tube).

'You'd best pack your bag,' she tells Serena. 'I'm pretty sure you will be off on the helicopter.'

It is a big deal for most of the families on the island to go to the mainland, let alone for Serena's family. To be sure she is not putting her to the expense and inconvenience unnecessarily, Adele sends her to Claris so that Ivan can give her a second opinion.

As it happens, Ivan has no hesitation in agreeing and the helicopter is summoned back to the island for its second mercy dash of the day.

The stoicism that in part alerted Adele to the seriousness of Serena's condition almost costs her dearly on the mainland. Once on the ground in Auckland, an ambulance takes her to the hospital, and when they arrive, it is to find that there are no wheelchairs.

'How far is it?' Serena asks. 'If it's not far, I'll just walk.'

The sight of a suspected ectopic pregnancy arriving on her own two feet makes the hospital staff sceptical; every other ectopic pregnancy they have ever seen has arrived groaning in agony on a stretcher. As she is sitting in her cubicle with the curtain drawn, Serena hears a doctor discussing her case on the phone.

'This is the second one we've had from the Barrier today. The last one did have an ectopic, but this one probably only has indigestion.'

A doctor puts in an IV line, and then Serena is left to her own devices for several hours. She goes to the toilet and faints, but recovers and returns meekly to her cubicle again. The second time she gets up to go to the toilet, bending over with the intense pain in her lower abdomen, she collapses again and this time, it is noticed. She is immediately rushed first for a scan and then straight into theatre.

'You and Ivan were right, Adele,' she says, upon her return a few days later. 'The scan showed an ectopic pregnancy and apparently, I had a litre of blood in my abdomen. They didn't waste the helicopter on me like they thought.'

Of course, hospital culture has changed since those days, and patients (and rural nurses) are treated with respect. Communication has improved out of sight—although getting quality information from the hardy islanders about the seriousness of their condition remains an art.

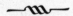

It is often noted that the concept of 'health' is different for people from rural areas and people from urban areas. In rural areas, people tend to think that if their body is performing the function they require it to perform—and mostly this equates to being up to whatever their work demands—then they are fit. You will look a long way before you will find too many of the 'worried well' people whom you might expect in any other community.

Back in the very early days before we were equipped with an X-ray machine, Adele and Ivan felt that orthopaedics—the diagnosis and treatment of musculoskeletal problems—was their Achilles' heel. In the absence of X-ray imaging, it was often difficult to tell whether a patient might need an expensive trip to Auckland.

One weekend, a young man presented to the nurse's cottage with a shoulder injury.

'I was riding my farm bike and I canned off and landed right on this part here. Something went pop in my shoulder.' He indicated the point of his shoulder.

He was very sore, and carrying the shoulder strangely. He could not raise his arm above shoulder level without severe discomfort, and there was also some distortion, with a lump visible at the end of his collarbone. Adele knew that something was wrong, but had no idea what or how serious it was. But as she was talking to the patient, she saw a man walking down the road whom she thought she recognised.

'Wait here, if you don't mind,' she told her patient. She jumped in her car and pursued the man down to the wharf.

'Excuse me,' she said, hurrying up to him. 'I'm sorry, I can't remember your name, but you're a doctor, aren't you? I recognise you from somewhere.'

'I am a doctor, yes,' he replied, much surprised.

'Sorry to bail you up like this, but I'm the nurse here. I've got a man in my clinic who has injured his shoulder and I wondered if you would be able to have a look at it and give me an idea of what the injury might be?'

'Well, I am a doctor—' he smiled— 'but I don't think I'll be much use to you. I'm an obstetrician.'

Suddenly Adele remembered where she knew him from. She

had met him when she was working as a midwife.

'I am here just about to meet a friend off the seaplane. He's an anaesthetist. He'll probably be able to help.'

Adele returned to the clinic, and soon after the sound of the seaplane was heard, the two doctors appeared at her door. Adele led them into the clinic, where they examined the local man's shoulder.

'This is a sprung AC, do you agree?' the anaesthetist said.

'Yes.' The obstetrician nodded. 'I am confident you're right. Shall we call a helicopter?' they asked Adele, who told them that she would discuss it with the local doctor.

Armed with a diagnosis, Adele had a way forward. She phoned Ivan, who consulted his orthopaedics textbook.

'Acromioclavicular joint separation,' Ivan read. 'Typically occasioned by impact on the back of the shoulder . . .'

He read out the clinical signs. Everything matched.

'Nothing much to be done for it,' he said. 'Put it in a sling and rest it. It might heal with a slight distortion, but this is cosmetic.'

Adele relayed this information to the patient.

'Would you like to go to Auckland so that they can X-ray it to confirm it?' she asked.

'No,' he snorted. 'If you reckon you know what's up, that'll do me.'

'You might be left with a bit of a lump there,' she said. 'Are you worried about what it looks like?'

The patient laughed. 'Of course not! So long as I can use it . . .'

These days, we have an X-ray machine (courtesy of the Great Barrier Island Community Health Trust), and Ivan is licensed to use it. Orthopaedics quickly became our forte over the years. We have had numerous orthopaedic cases to deal with.

'So,' he is fond of saying, as he examines people's X-rays, 'you've come to the Barrier for a break, then, have you?'

Sometimes, the islanders can take self-reliance too far.

'Ma's finally gone and done it,' says the voice on the other end of the telephone at 11.45 pm.

Adele fumbles for her torch and shrugs into her dressing gown. She goes downstairs so that she can turn on a light and have a conversation without waking Shannon.

'What happened?' she asked.

'She went out on to the back porch to pull the cord that turns off the generator and it broke. She tripped over on the concrete. I think she's broken her left hip because she can't get up and she says it's really hurting.'

Only on the island would a medical first responder be consulting a tide chart right now, but that is what Adele is doing. It's a 20- to 30-minute boat ride to Stellinmark, the property from which the call has come, and whether Adele will be able to get access will depend on the tide.

'Tide's low, isn't it?' she says.

'Yep,' Sven confirms. 'I can't get the boat out to come and get you. Do you think you could send the helicopter? It can land right in front of the house.'

Adele leans to look out at the sky. There's a full moon hanging low over the hills and silvering some high cloud. There's no wind whatsoever. It might be possible to get the helicopter in.

'I'll see what I can do about the helicopter,' Adele tells Sven. 'I'll come first myself. Make sure you keep your mum warm, and give her two paracetamol, if you've got them. Not too much water, though. They'll want her to have nothing in her stomach when she gets to hospital, just in case they want to operate. I'll be there as quick as I can.'

Adele phones a neighbour who has a fast launch and asks if he would mind running her down the harbour to Stellinmark. He doesn't hesitate to climb out of his warm bed, row out to his boat and bring it alongside the wharf to collect Adele. Meanwhile, St John confirms the helicopter will be despatched: control will contact Adele at Stellinmark for detailed directions and give her an estimated arrival time.

Adele dresses warmly and slips her gumboots on. She leaves a message for Shannon and changes the emergency message on the answerphone. Then she sets off. The launch is waiting at the wharf for her, the engine idling.

'Nice night for it, Adele,' the skipper says. Once she is aboard, he casts off, motors out into harbour, swings the bow to the south and opens out the throttle. The boat comes up on the plane, the spray shining phosphorescent in the darkness.

Adele knows her patient quite well. She always stood out—she was in her mid sixties when Adele first came to the island, and she would often come to Port FitzRoy for supplies for the remote farm on which she lives with Sven, her son. Adele would see her expertly bring her boat alongside the wharf, tie up and climb ashore, dressed in practical clothes—trousers and gumboots—but also giving off an air of sophistication with her makeup and jewellery. Adele has heard her story bit by bit over the years: her patient is the daughter of a wealthy Wellington businessman, is highly educated and accomplished. She married her cousin, Dion Stellin, who was expected to take over the running of the family business. But Dion seems to have been something of a wandering soul, and when he chanced upon the Barrier it captured him, as it has a tendency to capture such souls. He initially purchased Okiwi Station in 1957 and, when he judged the time was right, he brought his wife and three children over to join him.

She had no idea what to expect of the island. Perhaps she had been wooed by the stories Dion had told of his days on the islands of the Mediterranean during the Second World War, and in the Pacific and South East Asia since then. She told Adele that she wore her good dress and carried a parasol on the trip over. The Barrier was a culture shock! Sven says that when Ma arrived on the farm and Dion showed her the ramshackle, leaky homestead in which she and her three children were to live, she cried for two weeks. Her father was so horrified at the conditions into which her husband had dragged her that he withheld all financial support. Later, they purchased and moved to a property that was farmed by the Flinn family and occupied the peninsula at the southern end of Port FitzRoy harbour. Life was consequently hard, especially when Dion badly injured himself in an accident on the farm. She had to do all of the work in the house and on the farm—and all of the work was hard—but she coped, as islanders do. She was an accomplished equestrian, an avid reader and could hold up her end of a very sophisticated conversation. On Aotea, she added the ability to dig a garden, fish, operate a chainsaw and split firewood as well as muster sheep on horseback. But, once Dion was able to work the farm again, she took her children back to the mainland to complete their secondary schooling.

After finishing secondary school, Sven returned to the Barrier in 1973 to help his dad with the farm, which was just about completely overgrown with scrub. Instead, two years later, he found himself running the farm when Dion died of cancer. He was just nineteen. He received a bequest from his wealthy uncle and went, as he has put it, from being 'an impoverished, ignorant farm boy' to being 'a very wealthy, ignorant farm boy.' By his own admission, he made some questionable choices and soon ran through his money. His ma shifted over to help him with the house and the farm and to keep an eye on him. The two of them had been trying to make a go of it ever since.

—⁓—

Just after one in the morning, Adele and her boatman tie up at the jetty at Stellinmark. Adele clambers up a rickety steel ladder on their small wharf and walks up the path to Sven's house—the new home barged over after the Flinn homestead burned down in the family's early days—checking for tree limbs and overhead wires that will pose a hazard for the helicopter. She finds Sven watching over his ma, who is in a great deal of pain. She has been lovingly draped in blankets, and Sven has wrapped a shawl around her head, because it is a cold night.

'What have you done?' Adele asks her.

'Oh, I feel so silly,' she replies. 'I went to give a great big pull on the generator cord and it snapped. I lost my balance and fell on my hip.'

Adele examines her. It is clear she has indeed likely fractured the neck of her femur. She doesn't seem to have broken her wrist, which sometimes occurs when a hand is put out to break such a fall. Her blood pressure, pulse, respiratory rate and temperature are all satisfactory. Adele puts in an intravenous line so that she can administer some stronger pain relief.

The telephone is a relatively recent addition to Stellinmark, as the family re-christened the farm. Until quite recently, they had only a CB radio with which to stay in touch with the outside world. That would have added another layer of difficulty to this situation. Instead, Adele contacts St John and the control centre patch her through to the helicopter pilot, who is already in the air. She gives him the GPS coordinates from the boat's chart plotter and can assure him there are no landing hazards. Around 2 am, the throb of the rotors can be heard.

Adele and the paramedic who has accompanied the helicopter finish splinting the leg, and at 2.50 am, the helicopter lifts off for the trip to the hospital. Adele reassures Sven and gathers up her gear, clambers back down the rickety ladder, and the boat heads back up the harbour with the moonlight sparkling on the water. She is in bed again just before 4 am.

Now, one year on, the almost unprecedented situation has arisen where we are off-island completing postgraduate study in Dunedin. In order to be able to go, Adele has talked a colleague—a nurse and midwife—into standing in for her. She was nervous, but Adele assured her it was a quiet time of the year and that the others in the team would back her up.

Adele's cell phone goes just before we are about to go into a lecture.

'I've got some sad news, Adele,' her colleague says. 'Sven phoned. His mother died in her sleep last night.'

This is not unexpected, although sooner than we thought. She had been in gradual decline since returning from hospital. Our main focus has been palliative care. The nurse will have to attend, and the doctor from Claris will have to examine her and issue a death certificate. Adele phones Shannon to ask him to provide the necessary transport by boat.

A few hours later, her phone rings again.

'You won't believe this,' her colleague says, sounding panicky. 'I just went down to Stellinmark with the GP to do the death certificate. Sven says he's going to cremate his mother himself!'

Adele doesn't believe it, although she remembers all of the times that Sven has said, 'I'll just burn Ma up right here on the farm when the time comes', and she has laughed.

'Does he seem serious?'

'Well, he's out there with his bulldozer digging a hole, and he has a friend there stacking firewood beside it. I'd say he's serious!'

Adele phones Sven.

'I hear you're planning to cremate your mum. You're not really going to do that, are you?'

'Yes. That's my plan. Always said I would.'

'You know it's illegal, Sven, don't you?'

'Yes. Been reading up on it, Adele. The offence is called "interfering with human remains", and it carries a maximum penalty of a two-hundred-dollar fine.'

Adele tries a different tack, and explains that crematoria are specially designed to create a fire that reaches the fantastically high temperature you need to consume a human body. Try burning a body at a lower temperature, and the results could be horrific.

'You don't want those sorts of memories,' she says.

'No problem there, Adele,' Sven said. 'I've thought this through. I know we need a fire that burns between eight hundred and a thousand degrees. Well, I've got three tonnes of dry pūriri here, ready to go. Heat's not going to be a problem.'

Adele is feeling panicky herself, now. She is starting to run out of arguments.

'What do your sisters think of this idea?' she asks on a sudden inspiration.

There is a short silence on the phone.

'They're not here yet,' he says, sounding evasive.

Adele breathes a sigh of relief. Surely no daughter will allow her mother to be treated this way.

She stops worrying and, sure enough, she is present at an Auckland crematorium about a week later where there is a wonderful, packed farewell for Sven's ma.

A few months later, Adele asks Sven whether he thinks he might have been a bit manic after his mother died.

'No, not at all,' he says. 'Ma and I talked it over. It's how she wanted it.'

'What changed your mind? Was it your sisters?'

'No, it was the number of people who rang and said they really wanted to say goodbye to Ma but couldn't get to the island.'

Adele breathes a sigh of relief—but she has never been able to talk her colleague into relieving for her in the north of the island again.

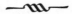

The islanders' need to be self-reliant exposes them to all sorts of risks that people on the mainland will never encounter—wind turbines that need servicing up ladders, and roofs that need to be climbed regularly so that solar panels can be cleaned. People have to walk streambeds collecting parts of their water turbine after yet another flood has demolished their micro-hydro scheme, or they have to shimmy past a chugging generator in a dark, shadowy shed . . . Heating water is often done the old-fashioned way, using a wetback on a wood stove. Having a soak in an outdoor bath heated by a wood fire underneath can be a heavenly experience, but it is not without its dangers. There is one case Leonie thinks of in particular where the daughter of a local rural fireman had returned to the island for a visit, and needed no persuasion to have a bath in the tub that her father had ingeniously contrived to heat with a safe firebox beneath the bath and a flue alongside it—a bit like a pizza oven with a bath perched on top. She had a lovely soak and felt thoroughly spoilt, but as she went to reach for her towel at the end of it, her delicate derrière made contact with the flue. She sustained serious burns to both buttocks—a painful reminder.

But Leonie has another story about the health risks that attend living off the main electricity grid.

Leonie takes the call. She quickly alerts Ivan and Peter.

'It's Richard,' she says, naming a man whose property is at the extreme southern end of Aotea. 'He has sustained a leg injury. Sounds very serious. He has told Patty that he has completely severed his foot on the fly-wheel of his generator.'

Ivan and Leonie race to their vehicle. They drive to rendezvous with the policeman, whom Leonie has summoned: his vehicle is also the local ambulance. The two vehicles quickly travel in convoy along the rough road to Richard's block. They park at the bottom of the steep track—and even by Aotea standards, this is a steep track—Ivan grabs his bag and sets off at a run, with Leonie and the policeman lugging emergency packs and struggling in his wake. It is early evening by now, and dark under the trees. They slip and stumble up the track: the policeman leads the way, but every now and again, he loses his footing and slips back towards—sometimes even past— Leonie. He blames his footwear; he has not yet broken in the tread on his new boots, he exclaims. Leonie is not too upset; the halts give her a chance to suck in a breath or two. Her footwear is sturdy: she is wearing her new Birkenstock sandals.

They finally reach the scene. Richard is sprawled outside the little shed that houses the generator, at a moderate distance from his house. Ivan is kneeling beside him, assessing the scene and surveying Richard's injuries by torchlight, and his friend is there, too, supporting, but looking pale and anxious.

Leonie lights her own torch to increase visibility. It shines on Richard's lower leg. She can see that the foot is completely disarticulated at the ankle. She closes her eyes momentarily. It appears to be merely hanging by an inch-wide skin tag to the rest of the leg. The distal—or bottom half—of the tibia is protruding through the stump, denuded of all but shreds of muscle and cartilage. The fibula appears to have been fractured and the skin at the bottom of his leg looks to be significantly contaminated with debris and is pale and devitalised. It is not a pretty sight, although it is better than she was expecting. Because she has not been in a war zone she has no experience in this kind of traumatic amputation, and nor has she previously been aware of the phenomenon of vasoconstriction, where the body reacts by reducing the arterial blood supply to amputated limbs. She had been expecting vast quantities of blood spattered around, pooling on the ground and gushing from the injury.

'I've made a bad blue,' Richard says, almost conversationally. 'I knew the key-way on the driveshaft of my generator had a sharp point on it. I was going to file it off, but—you know—it ended up being one of those round-to-it jobs . . . So I was in the shed, trying to do something to the genny, and the key-way gets hold of the trackies I was wearing. First I know about it, I'm rotating through the air and crashing into the machinery. The trackies were gone. *Oh bugger*, I thought. I tried to get up, but then I realised my foot was flapping around and I was standing on the bare knuckle of my ankle. Not good. So I hit the floor and dragged myself up on the door to yell to Patty.'

The first she knew of it, his wife confirms, was when Richard yelled, 'My foot's come off! You better call Ivan!'

Peter arrives, and that galvanises Leonie into action. Though he is stoic and his vital signs are stable, Richard needs medication to relieve the pain. Ivan needs to insert a large-bore angiocath into each of Richard's forearms. Peter is supporting the foot to keep patent (open) any surviving blood vessels to try to maintain the viability of the foot until we can properly dress and splint the limb.

'It's in,' Ivan says, having inserted the first angiocath. Leonie connects it to the fluid bag and asks someone to stand to hold it high to increase the flow. She turns to pick up the syringe of analgesia, but this occasions an unfortunate movement of her foot. The fancy side buckle of her Birkenstock catches the IV line and rips it out before Ivan can make it secure with tape.

Precious saline hoses on to the ground. Ivan looks at her impassively.

'Leonie, pass me another sixteen-gauge angiocath,' he says, and even adds 'please'. Leonie complies, and squats awkwardly, with an apologetic look on her face. She remains where she is until this second angiocath is in place, safe and sound.

More people arrive. It is the volunteer firemen, who are here to carry the stretcher. When Ivan judges him ready, Richard is lifted and carried carefully down the treacherous slope. Richard is six-foot-five (and a half) and is longer than the actual stretcher's capacity, and this concerns Ivan who is supervising from the rear. It is dicey on the dark, steep track, and inevitably one of the stretcher-bearers slips over. Richard lurches sideways. The others hastily counter-balance to rescue the situation. Richard is safe.

At the roadside, the sheer length of Richard creates problems. The stretcher cannot be clipped into its usual safety slots, because his splinted foot would protrude from the rear door. All kinds of frantic rearranging of the vehicle interior ensues, with jury-rigged restraints applied to the stretcher. It is not perfect but it's safe, and soon they grind off to the health centre to prepare for the helicopter and evacuation to Auckland Hospital. Finally, after the safety lights are positioned around the airfield, the helicopter lands.

Everyone is exhausted as they watch the winking lights of the helicopter recede into the inky blackness to the west.

Richard is back on the island eight weeks later. He has suffered several set-backs in his recovery, but now he has had a prosthesis fitted over the healed stump. At first, we were concerned about the remoteness of his situation and the uneven terrain he would have to negotiate every day, but his progress and stability has been rapid.

'Soon as I was home, I came right.' He grins. 'Once home, I never looked back.'

Home counts for so much. And for the islanders Aotea is home.

Chapter 11

NEARING
THE END

'It's a daunting privilege,' Professor Rod MacLeod, a palliative care specialist, writes in the introduction to *Snapshots: On the journey through death and remembrance*, 'to accompany people who are approaching death. One of the challenges is to balance the role of guiding and encouraging with the acknowledgment that people must travel the last part of the journey in a way that is uniquely theirs.'

No less than standing beside a mother as she gives birth, nursing a person as death approaches is a very sacred time. Often an intimacy is created within the circle of carers, and the rest of the world is somewhat closed off. The hallmarks of palliative care are seen as compassion and to alleviate suffering in order to secure the maximum possible quality of life and, ultimately, a 'good death'. The same palliative care specialist quoted above compares approaching death to walking along a mountain ridge. Factors beyond your control—the weather and the terrain—may affect the journey, and the final gate can be seen, first in the distance, but steadily drawing near. We have found this analogy helpful, because inevitably, as rural nurses, we have often been called upon to walk the journey besides people we know very well.

We all approach death in a different way. Just as we have learned to tailor births on the island to the individual woman's choices, so we have sought in every palliative situation to accommodate the wishes and needs of the patient along with those of their family. It is humbling to see how people approach this time—children willingly suspend their lives on the mainland or even further afield in order to become their parent's carer; partners—often frail and elderly themselves—spend hours just sitting holding their loved one's hand or snuggling up beside them on the bed. The same scenes are bound to occur on the mainland, but on the island, there is not the same access to the range of professional support services available elsewhere—the family is far more to the fore. It is almost unheard of for a Great Barrier Island patient reaching the terminal phase to choose (or to be compelled by family choices) to make the exhausting physical journey to a hospice. Generally speaking, it is just the family and friends caring, with the health team guiding, with increasingly frequent visits as death draws near.

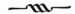

She is still the same gracious, wonderful woman we all know, even though she is in her nineties and the end is close. She has decided not to seek further investigations while at the hospital for her cancer-like symptoms. She has chosen instead to return to her island home until she dies.

'I know I have made the right decision,' she has said to Leonie several times. Even now that it is plain that the end is near, she is content.

Leonie is primly sitting in her beautifully appointed bedroom as they review her care. She herself is propped on a stack of plump pillows.

'Do you have pain?' Leonie asks.

'No, not really. I think it is really well controlled with those pills you arranged. But I've noticed I'm increasingly unsteady on my feet at night when I get up to use the commode. It's OK during the day when my helper is here. I do so appreciate her care, but I worry about it at night.'

Leonie wonders if there is anyone in the community she may be able to cajole into taking on night relief duties.

'I must admit, Leonie,' the woman says, 'it has gone on long enough. I was ready to go ages ago. I can't see the point of being on death's door for months.'

Leonie commiserates.

'I just wish it would hurry up. It is hard on my son. I don't think he is getting enough sleep. He's not as young as he once was, you know.'

They both laugh together. She listens to her patient's stout heart, and, while there are faint indicators of failure, the beat is steady and surprisingly strong.

As Leonie is putting her equipment away, the woman lowers her already hollowed-out voice to a conspiratorial whisper.

'Look at this, Leonie.'

She delicately throws back her covers and shows Leonie her 'pull-up' nappies. Against her tanned skin she has rolled the waistband down so that they are the shape of a bikini bottom.

'That is an improvement, isn't it?'

Leonie laughs out loud. It is typical of her patient—classy to the end.

She cheekily splashes some of her perfume on Leonie as she is about to go. 'This is one of my favourite scents. Have you smelled it before?' She shows Leonie the bottle. 'It suits you. It's called Joy.'

For a few weeks afterwards, even after the end has come for her patient, each time she gets in her car, Leonie fancies she can catch the lingering scent of Joy.

—m—

There is a short pause on the other end of the phone after Leonie has answered it. Then a voice choked with emotion says: 'Can you come now?'

Leonie has been expecting this call—perhaps not so soon, but even so, it is not a surprise.

She had a visit to this patient scheduled for this afternoon, but her instincts tell her something important is happening. She summons Ivan too, in case he is needed, and they climb into their car and head off.

It was only fifteen months ago that she and Ivan visited this man's home to inform him of the test results that confirmed an aggressive cancer. A mainland specialist had made the compassionate decision to ask Ivan to deliver the news to him on the island rather than to drag him across to the mainland, just to hear the tragic diagnosis. Their patient was a young man in his prime, a beloved husband and the adored dad of two daughters; in the aftermath of that terrible news, they all clung together and cried. Over the last fifteen months, his strong faith in God has clearly become his strength, sustaining him, and helping him along a difficult path: his palliative management has been challenging. His extended family and friends have supported him and his family wonderfully well every arduous step of the way.

At the top of the steep driveway, Leonie and Ivan get out of the car. The home has a stunning view over the beach: there have been many days, lately, where all their patient has wanted to do is gaze out the window at his beloved beach and the surf break where he has spent some of the best moments of his life—riding the waves, or simply walking in the squeaking sand hand-in-hand with his three girls.

They quietly let themselves in the ranch slider of his room. His wife is cradling him in their big double bed, and it is immediately obvious that his end is close. His breathing is laboured and shallow. Leonie quickly heads out through the house to fetch his daughters, and then she and Ivan step into the background. Soon afterward, surrounded by his family—his loving wife and his weeping daughters—his breathing slackens and then, finally, stops. He has slipped away from them to be with his Lord.

'Sorry to call you up here so suddenly,' his wife tearfully says. 'He didn't want me to be alone when it happened. He asked me to contact you. I just didn't realise that his death was so close.'

Outside, as they emerge from the room, Leonie gazes out over the beach far below. The waves are still rolling in from the broad Pacific, rearing as they near the land and breaking, casting themselves on the sand and then drawing back. As each wave spends itself, another is gathering behind it.

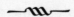

'Come in,' the woman says, her face streaked with tears. 'He's through here. He is not in a good way, I'm afraid. He's saying all sorts of stuff. Just so you know . . .'

Leonie is accompanied on this visit by one of the GPs from the health centre. They are here to see a man she knows very well. He is a colourful character, and his life has had more than its share of ups and downs. Leonie remembers grieving with him and his wife when their son died, twenty years ago. She remembers laughing with him over the antics of his grandchildren. She also remembers as though it was yesterday when he first presented with what he described as an annoying lump in his throat, and was referred to the mainland. He had reported recently that the oncologists had discovered another cancer. It was the second time he had faced the disease, and Leonie empathised with him as he contemplated another round of draining trips back and forth across the Hauraki Gulf to hospital stays and out-patient clinic appointments.

Leonie remembers the pang she felt when he told her that the surgeons had pronounced the disease inoperable. And today, she has learned that he has secondaries in his brain and that he has returned to the island. He is not expected to live long: perhaps no more than a few weeks.

His wife shows Leonie and the doctor through to his darkened room where the patient is lying in bed, his frame ravaged by the disease. They have with them some literature they give people when they are facing the end, mostly information about palliative care options and what to expect. It is a time to answer family questions and discover expectations so that they can guide his care. But the patient pre-empts them.

'There's got to be something you can give me to end all this. If I was an animal, they'd have put me down weeks ago,' he says.

Despite his wife's warnings, Leonie finds this brutal request unexpected. She feels tears spring to her eyes, and momentarily she does not know what to say. The GP remains by his bedside, quietly reassuring him and openly teasing out his fears. There is an intimacy in this moment—a time to leave his care in the GP's skilful hands.

Leonie puts her arm around her patient's wife's shoulders and leads her out of the room into the kitchen, where she slumps at the kitchen table as Leonie makes a pot of tea. The cup steams in front of the grieving wife as she sobs, head in hands, and Leonie tries to imagine the conversation in the bedroom.

Then, abruptly, the wife draws a deep, shuddering breath, dashes the tears from her eyes. She stands, smiling grimly at Leonie.

'Come and look,' she says mischievously. 'Just in case,' she adds.

Leonie is wary, trying to fathom this sudden change of mood. But she follows, and looks where indicated: in a high cupboard, she can vaguely make out a key tucked unobtrusively in the corner.

'He told me he didn't want me to be held responsible if he was found dead. This scared the living daylights out of me,' she says. 'So I took anything poison we might have and hid it. He'll never find the gun-safe key up there. Problem solved.'

Leonie is reeling with the implications of this when the GP appears, still wearing a wise, sad smile from her conversation with the dying man.

'Don't worry about what he is saying. It's a cry for help,' she says. 'It is quite understandable, really. He's afraid. He is afraid of the things you might expect him to be afraid of—pain, death—but he is also afraid of losing control and he is afraid of being even more of a burden on his family. All I've done is talk those fears through with him, and he is calmer now. We will need to be careful, but I think he's in a better space now. Leonie, he wants to talk to you now. He wants to be reassured that you can help his wife.'

Leonie returns to the bedroom and forces her own anxieties to the background while she simply listens as he pours out his anguish. The written material she brought to give to him she keeps to herself: it's superfluous. She knows that suffering comes in all guises, not merely the physical. This form of suffering is harder to palliate, but it is no less real.

Over the next few days, he settles back to his old self.

'He hasn't said anything like that again,' his wife says. She, too, seems steadier. She trained as a nurse, and her husband has asked her to take care of him in his last days. He really wants to die at home on the island, the place he loves best. This she has devoted herself to doing, supported by their amazing son.

The end when it comes a few short weeks later is peaceful and natural, and he is laid to rest in the Barrier's rich soil in a coffin lovingly crafted 'for the old bugger' by his son in their garage.

—⟋⟋⟋—

Leonie takes a deep, shuddering breath.

'I can't believe it,' says a stunned husband. 'Just an hour ago, she was so . . . alive. Now she's . . . gone.'

As they kneel together, the still, warm body of his wife lies on the floor between them, the marks of the sticky defibrillator pads still visible on her chest along with a warm pink tinge where hands have repeatedly tried to bring her back to life.

'It's all such a shock,' he says. 'She just got back from hospital . . . I thought she would be all right now.'

The GP has already removed the breathing tubes from her airway so that the husband can kiss and hug her one last time while she is still warm to his touch. Tears run freely down his face as he struggles to stand again. The newly arrived St John paramedic steps forward and takes him in his arms. They hug.

Leonie moves about, quickly gathering up the packaging and debris scattered beside the needle sharps container. It is time to remove all the medical paraphernalia before the rest of the woman's summoned family arrive.

Slowly, with time, the atmosphere settles. The rest of the health team have drifted back to work and the St John ambulance has returned to its depot. The husband has made his important phone calls, and a cup of tea has been pushed into his hand.

'Shall we lay her out together now? Is that all right?' Leonie asks him, and he nods.

After death it is our island practice to 'lay out' the patient. Together we encourage and assist family members or friends to wash the body and gather their favourite clothes. This has become a meaningful ritual for families to farewell someone they love—a completion, a caring act. It is also necessary, in the absence of a funeral director, that the body is carefully aligned or positioned before rigor mortis sets in so that it can later be placed in the coffin.

The woman's friend is quietly standing beside Leonie and has borne witness to the entire event. She is keen to help—a final gift of friendship.

Her husband quietly watches and directs as Leonie and the friend gather her newly purchased clothes.

'She was looking forward to wearing that skirt,' he says.

'Those are the knickers she would have wanted,' her friend adds. 'They were to be her special-occasion ones. I guess that's what this is.'

They all chuckle.

Leonie misses the daughter's presence. She is on the next plane and so cannot be part of the intimate circle yet. She will soon be here, along with her brothers and the wider family.

As her husband looks on, Leonie and the friend work to an age-old rhythm, washing and caressing her limbs and body. Like childbirth, it is an ancient ritual—women gathering to perform the tasks that are necessary. Both birth and death forge and strengthen the bonds that tie a community together.

They chat with her about all manner of things.

'Bad enough calling my gluten-free pastry "crap" that I especially made for you. But this is ridiculous.' Her friend half laughs, half sobs. 'She wasn't happy with my pastry treat,' she explains to Leonie. 'It had got stuck to the roof of her mouth. She's trying to unstick it and then next thing I know she's had a stroke and toppled over and taken me down with her. Really, it wasn't that bad!' she teases her friend. 'Did you have to go this far?'

With her body lovingly cleansed, Leonie and the friend dress her in the chosen clothes and stroke her face and brush her hair. Soon it is done, and everyone has taken their first step along the long road to acceptance.

'Thank you,' her husband says, as he hugs Leonie and the friend. 'She looks so peaceful.'

It is time now to greet the arriving family and friends.

Adele and Shannon are at the Port FitzRoy Boat Club. As usual, the men are down one end of the room, while the women are at the other.

'Your husband's just had an argument,' someone says to Adele.

'What?' she says. 'Who with? What over?'

It turns out the storekeeper—Serena's granddad—has bailed Shannon up and told him his chickens have been scratching up his garden. Adele inherited the chooks from Fay: they were kept in a small run at the back of the nurse's cottage. But when Adele and Shannon moved to their new house a couple of kilometres down the road, the chooks remained. They have become a bit feral and instead of their chookhouse, they are roosting in the mānuka and, it seems, raiding the storekeeper's garden.

Adele looks around for Shannon, but he is nowhere to be found. She drives to the nurse's cottage and finds him standing under the mānuka, trying to coax the chooks down with a broom. They are not having a bar of it. Each time he swishes the broom, they cluck and flutter a little higher in the tree. Soon they are well out of broom range and simply ignore him.

('Did he use fowl language?' Ivan typically asks, when he hears about the episode later.)

'What would you do if you got them down, anyway?' Adele asks Shannon.

'I'll wring their necks and hang them outside the shop. That will sort them out.'

Adele persuades him that this might be a problem best tackled in the morning. The next day, they resurrect an old cage at their house and move the chickens into new accommodations with their necks intact, ensuring the storekeeper's garden is safe from their marauding and the family's friendship with Adele and Shannon is preserved.

Some time after this incident, and soon after he has embarked on what he has been hoping will be a long and fulfilling retirement, Adele is distressed to learn that the storekeeper has been diagnosed with terminal cancer. His wife is determined to nurse him, and Adele assumes the role of supporter to her, the primary caregiver, stepping in each time his disease enters a new phase and intervention is required. Sometimes, she calls at the house to listen; other times, she offers advice and reassurance, and more often than not, she does little more than have a cup of tea and sit in companionable silence with her friend and his family. On a couple of occasions towards the end of his six-month decline, they call her out at night, and she brings her sleeping bag to the house. But they always insist she return to her own home, and she finds herself crying as she drives home, remembering how supportive of her they had been, and the parts they have played in each other's lives these last twelve years.

As the end approaches, he tells Adele that he would rather she was present when he passes, as he does not want his wife to be alone. Consequently, one Friday afternoon, Adele is there when her friend gently slips from this life and ends his long struggle with his disease. She feels privileged to have been there and to be able to perform a last caring act, bathing him and laying him out on his bed dressed in his favourite clothes. It is Ivan's day off, but he willingly comes over to share in this day of sorrow and to begin to prepare for the service at which he will officiate. Telephone calls are made, and family, friends and food begin to arrive.

On Saturday, the shopkeeper's son-in-law and two friends dig a grave in the old private cemetery, in a grove of trees near a stream. Another son-in-law borrows a van to pick up the coffin made to order by a local artisan—it is of oiled macrocarpa, and smells of the bush. In the afternoon his son, a close friend and Adele lift him into the coffin and settle his favourite beret on his head. Here, according to Barrier custom, he is visited by friends and family as they gather to mourn and to be thankful for the life he lived.

On Sunday afternoon, Adele gives a woodscrew to Serena and to each of the man's three other grandchildren and to his two children, and they sadly use these to close the lid. The coffin is then taken to the garden of a friend to celebrate his interesting life. Afterwards, as he is laid to rest, Adele thinks of a few lines from a favourite John Masefield poem, 'By a Bierside':

> *Death makes justice a dream, and strength a traveller's story.*
> *Death drives the lovely soul to wander under the sky.*
> *Death opens unknown doors. It is most grand to die.*

No more than year later, her friend's house is sold to a young couple, and Adele finds herself assisting at the home birth of their third child. Ka pō, ka ao—it is night, it is day. The cycle continues.

One aspect of rural nursing that our careers have borne out is that, as a rural nurse, you are not so much serving the community as participating in it. You are part of the lives of the people among whom you live. Inevitably, this means that we have a lot to do with the tangata whenua: everyone who has come to live on the Barrier finds themselves more or less enfolded in the rhythms of taha Māori. The very first Pākehā who came here—the whalers, the bushmen, the gumdiggers—vitally depended on the tangata whenua, and, for their part, Māori often worked alongside Pākehā, participating in the new way of life that the Pākehā brought. This laid the foundations for the way of life that we have on the island today, where community is at the heart of things, and there is a strong sense of the importance of ritual in the lives of the people. There is a holism about the Māori perspective that aligns well with the ethos of nursing, and with rural nursing in particular.

Leonie is of Waikato-Tainui descent. And of course, many of our patients—approximately nineteen per cent—are Māori. The tangata whenua, Ngāti Rehua—Ngāti Wai ki Aotea whakapapa back to some of the earliest people in Aotearoa. It has been a joy and privilege for us to share part of their life journey.

—m—

The whare stirs Adele each time she drives into Motairehe. It is a white weatherboard bungalow with a back porch and a front verandah. It had been shipped to the island to replace an old whare that burned down. It is beautifully situated with the river on one side and the glittering waters of Katherine Bay spread out before it. Adele grew up in houses just like it: it reminds her of her childhood, and it holds other memories, too. Even now, Adele hasn't quite got used to the sight of the empty porch. A few years ago, it was the home of the sister of the man she's going to see, and it seemed she was always there to call out.

'Where are you off to, Adele? Is someone sick? Or are you here to see the babies?'

Each time Adele stopped to talk to her, she would come away with a new collection of stories about the people and the place around them.

Adele remembers the day she first looked for her on the porch and missed her.

She was inside, lying peacefully on her bed in the lounge. Like all these older New Zealand houses with their high ceilings and their lack of insulation, this one was cold in winter. Her whānau had installed a woodburner for her in the lounge and she had taken to sleeping there in that warm place. Her sisters were gathered at her bedside, along with other whānau. Her son was upset. He had been outside that afternoon mowing the lawns, and by the time he came in that evening to check on her, she had passed away. She was lying there, her Rātana Bible open on the bedside table to the last verses she had been reading.

'I should have been here,' her son said. 'She shouldn't have been alone.'

'No, you couldn't have been doing a thing better,' Adele consoled him. 'She went to sleep knowing you were close by and doing something for her.'

Still, he cried, and Adele cried too. Everyone cried and mourned the loss of a mother, grandmother, sister, aunty, mentor and friend.

She was the first. All three of the sisters who were at the bedside that day have gone to be with her now. And now it is their brother's turn to pass on.

⬥

Adele and her colleague Denise wait solemnly with a number of others at the waharoa (entrance place), quietly talking among themselves. Across the road, in a haze of smoke from the hāngī fire, is a group of young men with shovels and piles of dirt—preparations are underway for the hākari (feast) to be held later.

'OK,' someone says. An indication has been given that all is ready and the group tightens up, wāhine in front and tāne at the side and towards the rear.

'Haere mai rā, haere mai, haere mai . . .'

A karanga rings out inviting the manuhiri—the visitors—on to the marae. The caller, the kaikaranga, stands dressed in black, fluttering her hands. The woman who has been appointed kaiwhakautu (the senior woman among the visitors) stands out in front of the manuhiri and replies: 'Karanga mai, karanga mai, karanga mai . . .' and the manuhiri walk slowly forward. It is an ancient ritual, with every word and movement replete with meaning, tying the present generation to the past, the living to the dead. It is a human cycle to match the natural cycle to which we are all subject. Adele feels the welling of emotion that she always feels during the karanga. It is always such a spiritual moment.

The manuhiri pause at the door and there is a shuffling as everyone takes off their shoes. They walk slowly across the whāriki (woven mats), past the tangata whenua along the walls of the house. Adele stops for a moment, remembering her own father, as well as all the people to whom she has previously bid farewell on this marae and pays a quiet tribute to the tūpāpaku (body) before her. Then she moves on to greet the whānau pani (bereaved family). Some she knows well. Some she knows rather less well, or not at all.

She pauses beside the casket and addresses the man lying within it, his face made gaunt by illness but relaxed in his final rest. As is the custom, Adele says her last words to the dead man, in the belief that his wairua (spirit) lingers and will hear her.

'They've brought me home to die,' he had said when Adele dropped in to visit him. He had been a tall, well-built man, and although cancer had diminished him, stripped the weight from him, the spark of his humour was still all there. 'They reckon I'm going to die, but I'm not, you know.'

'Glad to hear it,' laughed Adele.

In spite of his defiance, they both knew he was terminal. He had been sick for a long time and was on palliative care back in Auckland before his whānau decided it was time to bring him home. Adele was sad, because he was the last of his generation. The girls—his sisters—had all gone.

One summer's Saturday afternoon, he phoned. 'You know, Adele, there are all these young folk kicking a ball around on the beach. None of them will help me mow my lawns or get firewood. What's wrong with this generation?'

'I'm your nurse, not your social worker,' Adele replied. 'Don't complain to me, because I can't even get one of them to help me wash my car. Anyway, they're probably too scared, because they know they couldn't do it to your standards.'

They both laughed.

By the time he had begun his final decline, it was winter and cold outside. Yet the interior of his house was filled with the warmth of love and caring. He was content. A nephew dropped in regularly with his favourite food: kina, mussels, oysters and fish. Each time Adele visited, she found him beautifully groomed and snugly wrapped in blankets, sitting up on his La-Z-Boy chair. He had no need of drugs: he was cocooned in aroha and surrounded by his whānau.

After a hymn and karakia, the whaikōrero starts—always first acknowledging the Creator, the whare, the earth mother, the marae, the first caller of the day (the kaikaranga), the dead (the ancestors behind the veil)—before moving on to the living and the most recently dead. The speakers intersperse humour with their oratory. The laughter is a relief from the sadness, the sadness is a reminder that there is sorrow amidst all the joys of life. After each speaker, people get to their feet and a waiata is sung. The sound of the singing is beautiful and uplifting.

Adele is not fluent in te reo. She can follow some of what is said, but does not try too hard. She is content to be lulled by the sound of this poetic language and the answering murmurs of the listeners. And as she half listens, she looks towards the photos that are propped up around the coffin, reminders of the whānau now deceased. With a mild shock, Adele reflects that when she first came to the island, she didn't know who any of these people were. Now, after all this time, many of the people in the photos are known to her, and the photos bring back vivid memories. She realises that she is rapidly becoming a part of that older living generation herself.

At the end of the speaking, there is a final, loud outpouring of grief. The casket, Adele knows, is being closed. Soon it is carried by, and Adele too cries as he passes.

A procession forms behind the casket. For his sister's burial, the walk to the urupā (cemetery) entailed a long walk across the creek, along a treacherous track around the point, whereupon everyone would have to pick their way up the steep track that climbs the mountain behind the next bay. Everyone made that long, arduous walk behind their caskets, and on each occasion, Adele used to pack heart and respiratory emergency medications in her backpack for this journey in case any of the mourners fell by the wayside. They never did. The views from the top out over the bay are breathtaking. The urupā is surrounded by a white picket fence, with some very old head-stones marking the graves of previous generations who have been laid to rest there. On this day, everyone follows the whānau up the hill at the back of the marae to a newer, more accessible urupā. It is still a little demanding: even though the clay path has been overlaid with pine needles, Adele is glad she wore her gumboots.

The graves here descend the gentle hillside. He is to lie in peace at the top with some of his sisters and other family members, gone before, flowing down the hillside below. There are flowers, gentle sobbing, a rousing haka and finally karakia, a blessing and waiata. Everyone files past the open grave and acknowledges the whānau pani, then slowly makes their way back down the hill, pausing to wash their hands at the gate. Everyone sits on the grass back on the marae, talking and waiting to re-enter the wharenui for the final blessing. After that, the hākari will follow.

As one of the speakers eloquently put it: 'Kua hinga te tōtaranui o Te Waonui a Tāne' (a great tōtara has fallen in the sacred forest of Tāne). He was instrumental in building and maintaining the wharenui, where he lay and from which the final journey of his body began. He was also instrumental in building and maintaining his community, and he will live on in the people who are gathered here in his honour, too. These are the legacies he has left behind: the wharenui and the people.

Māori traditions have been woven into the warp and weft of community life on Aotea, and this is nowhere more obvious than in our attitudes towards dying and the rituals after death, how the body is cared for by the family and the 'form' of a Barrier funeral. Family members coming from off-island often remark on the positive difference in the way we do things, and they are almost always approving and appreciative of that difference. They experience being drawn into the community through the 'ties of love, respect and sorrow' as they mourn. This is what happens in the traditional tangihanga, and in our own, acculturated version of it. It is common that, when someone dies, they lie in state within the family home. Family and friends visit and share stories about the person's life. It is a time of being surrounded. The funeral gatherings are open community occasions when everyone draws together to celebrate the life of the person who has died. To tell anecdotes, pay tribute and express their grief with other mourners, bringing real comfort to the family. This is a time of strengthening relationships and creating interconnectedness.

While Barrier funerals are creative, so too are other aspects that lead up to the day. There are no actual funeral directors on Aotea, so the health team are charged with caring for the body until burial. In years past, there was pressure on families to create a coffin quickly as well as to assemble a team to dig the grave by shovel. There have been memorable coffins: friends of a local who died without on-island family took the dinghy he was building and created a lid to seal his remains inside. The coffin arrived at the graveyard on the back of a fire truck, flanked by Rural Fire Force volunteers and with the fire chief helmet that the community had given him on his eightieth birthday proudly affixed. In another, the owner of a building supplies company was laid to rest in a coffin fashioned to look like a 'packet' of timber. Families sometimes adorn the coffins with artwork and words of farewell. On the death of his partner, a local contractor had his own coffin made to match. It stood in their bedroom for years: he knew it would come in handy, sooner or later.

Transporting bodies to Auckland for cremation used to be problematic—there is little that can be done to disguise a police-issue black polythene body bag. In the mid-nineties, the Health Trust asked a local wood sculptor/artisan/builder to build coffins for emergency use, so he added 'coffin-maker' to the long list of his other occupations. The beautiful streamlined, unadorned casket he devised—one size fits all, and with carved wooden handles—has become known as 'the Barrier Coffin' and soon became the thing to use when someone died on-island. There have even been occasions when a Barrier Coffin has been shipped to the mainland on the request of off-islanders. Occasionally the plain coffin is personalised with additions, such as hoarded kauri pieces, lovingly carved, but it is most often the interior that is customised, with quilts or special blankets over the hygienically sealed base. The ritual screwing down of the lid by family members and friends is part of the farewell journey.

Aided by the Ngāti Rehua—Ngāti Wai ki Aotea, Ivan—partly because of his public health role as general practitioner, but also partly as a funeral officiant—assiduously lobbied for a proper mortuary. His main concern was for the tangata whenua—how much time and money was involved in sending a body to the mainland for embalming so that it could be returned and laid in state for tangihanga. It was also quite common for funerals to be delayed while off-island family made arrangements to come across for the funeral, and in hot weather this could be problematic, in the absence of somewhere cool.

Auckland City Council agreed and built a discrete three-room mortuary: an embalming room equipped with a chiller, a room where family may sit and be with the departed and a garage space for an ambulance or funeral hearse. It is from this mortuary, nestled among mānuka trees a short distance from the aerodrome, that caskets set off for the marae or their final resting place—when they are not lying in the deceased's home. We have never felt the lack of a purpose-built hearse: in fact, all types of vehicles have served in this capacity, including the four-wheel-drive health team vehicles. Often ferns will be laid beneath the coffin, and flowers laid on top. The trip to the graveyard is usually the shortest leg of a journey that may have begun weeks, months, even years before. It is a time in which the families have reflected on their own relationships and have needed support. There is an interconnectedness of life in such a small community— members passing down knowledge and skills, helping each other. It has been our privilege in so many cases to have made this journey alongside the islanders, shoulder to shoulder with others.

Chapter 12

BOLTS FROM THE BLUE

The medical and nursing councils give clear advice on treating those close to you, especially family members. But as health professionals on an island, Ivan and Leonie had to decide in the early days whether one of them would leave the island for the 24-hour turn-around with a sick child when there were many people unwell in the waiting room who needed immediate care. As tempting as it might be to bring your skills and training to bear when family members are involved, the recommendation is that you consult another GP colleague. Even Ivan has his own off-island general practitioner. So much for the biblical instruction: physician, heal thyself!

—⚒—

Leonie is working alone in the health centre when the phone rings. Her heart skips a beat when she hears her daughter's name mentioned on the other end.

'It's Amiria,' the wavering voice says. 'Her face has been ravaged by a dog.' That caught Leonie's immediate attention. 'Cherie is on her way.'

An image of her daughter's face, the smooth skin glowing with health, flashes before Leonie's mind's eye, but she banishes it.

She takes what details she can, hangs up and takes a deep, steadying breath.

She phones Ivan at the nurse's cottage, where he is conducting the Port FitzRoy Clinic. They talk briefly, and he is on his way, abruptly leaving the last patient to Adele. Then there is nothing to do but wait.

For some reason, although Cherie lives on the beach not far from the health centre, the wait seems interminable. A car finally arrives. Leonie is outside to meet it, and she gets her first look at Amiria's bloodied face. There is so much blood it is initially difficult to determine the extent of her injuries. Leonie is calm, partly because this is how she is trained to be, and partly because she needs to be for her daughter's sake.

As they go inside, she learns that a gaggle of children were eating a batch of Cherie's raisin buns, fresh from the oven, when a visiting dog ambled over for his share. Amiria was just taking a bite of her bun when the dog leaped at it.

Most of the blood seems to be coming from the vicinity of Amiria's right eye. Leonie begins to clean it away with sterile gauze, and discovers that there is thankfully only a small puncture wound in the white of her eye and a gash beside her eye. It is bleeding freely, but on superficial inspection both do not seem serious.

She keeps the relief at arm's length, just as she had earlier controlled her fear, but she finds it easier to perform the methodical tasks—cleaning the wounds and directing Amiria to keep pressure on the wound while she herself assembles the equipment she will need to suture the gash and perform a more thorough inner eye examination.

There is the sound of a vehicle arriving at speed. Leonie has forgotten about Ivan! A car door bangs, and Ivan bursts through the back door of the centre. He is pale, and his eyes are still wild with the adrenaline of his frantic hoon from Port FitzRoy. He will always describe this as the worst journey on the island he has ever made. In the absence of cell phones, at this time, Leonie could not allay his fears en route.

Leonie goes to brief him—one health professional to another—but suddenly the mum in her will be denied no longer. She bursts into tears.

In an ideal world, Ivan would allow someone else to review Amiria's eye injury and do the suturing of the small wound, but he is the only doctor on hand. He does it, although he phones a doctor on the mainland to seek moral support. There is no damage to the eye, and the only faint risk is from infection, which is easily averted with antibiotics.

For her part, Leonie is left shaking with relief and reflecting on how vulnerable we are on our isolated island. As nurses, we are trained to be objective and unemotional: she has coped, but she knows she will be haunted by that first glimpse of her daughter's bloodied, 'ravaged' face.

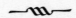

'Ivan.'

Leonie is sure she has heard something. She is busy preparing dinner, but something like a voice has intruded on her consciousness.

She looks out of the front door, but there is no one there. She listens hard, but hears nothing further.

Then Ivan puts his book down and looks out the window, frowning.

'Did you hear anything?' he asks Leonie. 'I think I heard someone calling out.'

He opens the door again and has a look outside. Nothing but the hiss and suck of cicadas in full throat: it is high summer—New Year's Day is only a few days hence—and the sun is blazing outside.

'Oh well,' he says, shrugging. 'Must be imagining things.'

We both jump as there is a loud blast on a vehicle horn. It is from the other side of the house, where the garage is. Ivan looks out and sees a ute parked there, and even as he looks, the driver's door opens and a man topples in slow motion on to the lawn.

He and Leonie rush out. It is Greg, one of the locals.

'What's going on, Greg?' Ivan asks, kneeling next to him.

'Throwing up . . . pooing . . .' Greg groans, and then mysteriously adds, 'John Dory.'

He retches violently, but only thin, yellow bile comes up.

Greg lives by the beach, and naturally he enjoys nature's bounty in the form of the abundance of kai moana that is on his doorstep. He loves mussels and pāua, and he fishes for snapper. But he has learned the hard way that some seafood doesn't agree with him. If he eats kahawai, he experiences nausea and vomits. He is wary of trevally, tarakihi, scallops and (there is always a note of regret in his voice when he says so) crayfish.

This morning out fishing, he caught his first ever kuparu (John Dory). These are very good eating, and he was looking forward to sharing it with friends who were coming over. Everyone agreed it was delectable.

It was only 90 minutes later, as he was arriving at the sports club, where he was to play tennis against a friend, that he began to regret eating the fish. His opponent arrived to find Greg leaning against the wall of the building and being violently sick.

'Gee, you're in no state to play tennis,' his friend said.

'No, sorry, mate,' Greg panted. 'Tennis is off.'

'You poor sod,' his friend said. 'Will you be OK?'

'Oh, it'll settle down,' Greg said.

But after his friend had driven away, it became clear that Greg's reaction to a protein in the fish was escalating. His head was whirling with nausea, and to make matters worse, he now found himself with a violent need to defecate. The sports club toilets were locked, so Greg hurried into the bushes nearby. He just managed to get his shorts down and to squat when his guts cramped and he emitted a stream of diarrhoea. Cramp after cramp assailed him, and he passed out.

When he came to—he had no idea of how much time had passed—he was weak and confused. There was no let-up in the bouts of vomiting, and his bowel was still cramping. But he knew he could not stay where he was. He knew he needed urgent medical attention.

Ivan, he thought.

He struggled to his feet, yanked up his shorts and stumbled, doubled over with abdominal cramps, to his ute. Somehow he managed to drive to the Howies' place.

Leonie and Ivan get this story in fragments, as Greg is in a bad way. He is pale, clammy and in a state of collapse. His vital signs are worrying: his pulse is fast and weak and his blood pressure is low. He is plainly grossly dehydrated and in shock.

After administering initial first-line treatment medications, Ivan and Leonie manhandle Greg into his ute and Ivan drives it rapidly up the road to the health centre. It is late afternoon but still very hot, and the stench makes Ivan gag, too. And when they arrive at the health centre, it is shut up and the interior temperature is sweltering. Leonie sets about opening every door and window to try to cool the place down quickly: the last thing Greg needs in his state is to bring on vasodilation—the widening of his capillaries as a response to the heat.

'Were you in the shower before you came?' Leonie asks Greg, but he shakes his head. He is literally bathed in sweat.

Between them, Ivan and Leonie have already established two IV lines and have begun administering saline to try to reverse Greg's dehydration. But as quickly as they can infuse fluids, his blood pressure drops, and drops, and drops.

'His chest is clear,' Ivan reports, listening with his stethoscope. 'And there is no sign of rash or angioedema. It is just the gastrointestinal and cardiac systems involved. Best try to contact anyone else who ate the fish, just in case this is a toxic reaction.'

In between assisting Ivan, Leonie gets on the phone. She learns that no one else has been affected. This is a relief, in some ways: instead of dealing with the effects of an unknown toxin, they are dealing with an allergic reaction. But still Greg's blood pressure falls. Ivan supplements the saline with extra volume expanders—it is possible to survive major dehydration as long as the blood pressure can be maintained so that oxygen still reaches vital tissues, and volume expanders assist in this.

'Still falling,' Leonie tells Ivan. She speaks calmly and precisely, and he answers in kind. Each knows their role intimately and they work together efficiently and purposefully.

They have infused nearly three litres of fluids: the circulatory system of your average adult male contains approximately five litres of blood. They are also nearing the maximal doses suggested in the primary context (that is, outside a hospital) of the drugs they are using.

'What do you think?' Ivan asks Leonie. Together, they review their protocols: what may be tried, what they have tried, and the rapidly diminishing options available to them.

'My head,' says Greg weakly. 'My head's killing me.'

'I'm afraid that's a side-effect both of dehydration and of the treatment,' Ivan tells him.

Leonie checks her watch. The emergency fixed-wing evacuation plane is still a long way off. The fluid is pouring off his skin, and he is clammy to touch.

'I feel better,' Greg says. 'I feel super calm.'

Leonie looks at Ivan. 'What does that mean?' she asks.

He shrugs.

'I'm drifting away,' Greg announces.

Ivan phones Accident and Emergency to seek further advice from the emergency physicians.

'Not much you can do but keep tipping in the fluids and the expanders,' they say. 'And repeat the meds. You've got to keep his pressure up. We're preparing for his arrival.'

That sounds ominous.

Leonie has replaced the bag of fluid twice, and a fifth litre begins trickling into his arm.

'It's really peaceful,' Greg says. 'I'm not worried at all.'

It dawns on Leonie that they really are losing him. She checks her watch. Each minute on the dial equates to tens of kilometres of empty ocean between themselves and onrushing assistance. She is conscious that panic is not far away, so she redoubles her efforts to concentrate on the tasks at hand. She checks his vital signs again.

'Greg's blood pressure, though low, is stabilising, Ivan,' she reports. 'His pulse is improving too.'

She checks again five minutes later, and sees with relief that it has even risen a little. Time is slowly passing.

'Do you have one of those bottle things?' Greg asks. 'I really need to pee.'

Leonie looks at Ivan and they grin at one another, relieved. Greg isn't out of the woods yet, but the need to urinate is a sign that his bodily fluid volumes are normalising and his kidneys are being perfused.

'I feel extremely super calm,' Greg says again.

Neither Ivan nor Leonie know how to interpret these statements. It is certainly not something they can recall from their text books.

The welcome buzz of the aircraft engines is heard, and soon the Great Barrier Island Airlines plane bounces to a stop on the airstrip—a welcome sight. A St John paramedic joins them and they update him on Greg's condition. He is satisfied he is stable and ready to evacuate, and it pleases the pilot that they can turn around quickly, too: he has been called away from the bedside of his wife, who is about to have a baby. When the plane finally lifts off into the sky, lights flashing, it is nearly dark. It has been three hours since the drama began. We are both physically and mentally exhausted, but we are pleased with the outcome. Thankfully, Greg's body has weathered this storm.

'Good work, Ivan,' Leonie says.

'Good work, yourself,' he replies.

We are having a lunchtime meeting at a cafe away from the health centre. It is a rare event because we have been able to align the windows in our schedules. Leonie is showing off her brand-new, cosy, wool-lined ankle boots, and Adele is suitably admiring.

The phone rings and Leonie is called by the cafe owner to take an emergency call, alerting her to a small plane crash in the swamp nearby. Then a man in the airline's uniform walks into the cafe with a small forehead gash. It is the co-pilot, and he tells us that after take-off the plane veered off into the raupō swamp just 400 metres from where we are standing. We swing into action.

The health centre is positioned beside the Claris Airfield and we have practised for such scenarios. This time it is for real. We quickly assign roles. Leonie will rush to the scene and triage—identify the most seriously injured—and Adele will assess and care for the co-pilot, return to the health centre to alert everyone there, assemble the vehicles as stand-by ambulances and return to assist with transporting the survivors—everyone on board, the co-pilot assures us.

'We lost power and the pilot put the plane down as gently as he could. We landed level but we hit pretty hard. Some of the passengers are badly injured.'

He gives as many details as he is able as they drive. He directs Adele to a point in the road that he thinks is closest to the crash site. Leonie straps on her backpack containing emergency gear and sallies forth into the raupō as Adele drives off back down the road towards the health centre.

Leonie strikes trouble immediately. The raupō is a lot taller than her: she feels like Minnie Mouse in the lush, green fastness of the swamp, and cannot orientate herself. She feels a rising panic when there is the sound of a labouring two-stroke motor out on the road. She hurries back to the roadside, and is grateful to see one of the taller locals puttering along on a diminutive motor scooter.

'Leonie!' he says. 'What are you doing in there? Do you need a hand?'

'I sure do!' she replies. 'There is a plane down in there, but I can't see where I'm going. Would you take this for me?' She gives him the heaviest emergency backpack. 'Lead the way!'

He obligingly stomps off into the swamp and Leonie follows as closely as she can, the brackish, far-from-fragrant water up to her thighs in places. The rushes close behind him quickly, so that she is claustrophobically walled in by the raupō. But she can hear his progress, and she follows the sound.

The crunching and the crashing stops after they have ploughed about 100 metres into the swamp.

'Over here!' he calls.

Leonie follows his voice and emerges from a wall of raupō into a clearing gouged by the plane. The plane itself is intact and resting on its belly, steam rising from the engines in the swamp. With a bit of help from her trailblazer, Leonie scrambles on to a wing and from here can assess the passengers in the fuselage. Some appear mildly shocked but otherwise OK, but it is clear two of them are seriously injured.

Leonie hears the sounds of other people making their way through the raupō, and she is relieved they will have help to extricate the injured. The emergency services have swung into action, and soon there is barely any room on the wing. The GP arrives with more emergency gear. The local roading contractors have assembled parties to stretcher out the two injured, and they are carefully secured in the scoop stretchers and slung down to waiting hands.

Leonie and the general practitioner follow a patient each out to the road where four-wheel-drive vehicles are waiting to convey them to the health centre. It is far easier walking out than it was walking in: the various sets of feet that have trodden down the raupō have created a veritable highway, and Leonie can walk on the flattened rushes without sinking into the mire.

Once the two serious cases are on their way, Leonie returns to assist with escorting the remaining passengers to the health centre for a fuller assessment. She finally stands in the nurse's station, dripping and decidedly not smelling her best. She ruefully tugs off her new boots—they come off with a squelch. She is glad she had them—they likely protected her from shredding her feet on sharp sticks and stones in the swamp—but they have paid the ultimate price.

She drops them in the wastepaper basket with a clang.

'So much for my lovely new boots!' she says. 'I think I will invest in steel caps next time.'

Everyone laughs, perhaps a little louder than necessary; the adrenaline has to be worked through one way or another.

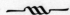

Leonie is baking with Amiria and Jordan. They are laughing and enjoying one another's company and Leonie is marvelling—as every parent marvels from time to time—at how big and capable they are getting. Then the phone goes. It is a neighbour of Jill's.

'She's collapsed,' he says.

'Is she conscious? Breathing?'

'Yes, she's breathing, but she's unconscious.'

Leonie puts down the phone, and she is in nurse mode. Mother mode has to wait. The children are used to this, and they carry on measuring and stirring as Leonie races to put on her sturdy walking shoes and shrugs into the straps of her backpack.

'Listen to see if the cake is talking when the buzzer goes,' she tells Ivan, who has put down his book and rolled up his sleeves ready to help with the baking. 'That recipe usually needs a few minutes longer, so be prepared to leave it in for another five minutes,' she calls as she races out of the room.

But even as she speaks her mind is already in professional mode, already running through scenarios and marking off items she may need on a mental checklist. She phones the new locum general practitioner and arranges to meet her en route. They will need her large four-wheel-drive to tackle the track to Allom Bay: her husband will drive—he is very skilled. With all organised, she climbs into her vehicle and sets off for the rendezvous.

After meeting up, they drive for twenty minutes along a track that gets steeper then narrower as it drops down into Blind Bay towards the west coast. At the road's end, they can see the water through the trees and then drive down on to a sandy beach. Another of Jill's neighbours is waiting there with a quad bike, which Leonie and the GP load up with their gear. The neighbour sets off with the GP perched uncomfortably behind him, and Leonie jogs along behind, struggling to keep up. It is fifteen minutes up then down through the bush to Allom Bay, around the point from the road-end. When she is getting close, she hears the approach of the prearranged Auckland Rescue Helicopter. When she breaks out into the open, on to the grassy flat adjacent to the foreshore where the small cottage that Jill rents out to guests is situated, she can see the big, red machine hovering, scoping a suitable place to land on the foreshore.

On closer inspection, in front of her she can see the cottage and Jill sprawled on the ground near the door, her children—her daughter is eight now, and her son six—huddled beside her. But there are two people she doesn't recognise—off-islanders—standing uncertainly in the background, too.

This moment will replay and replay with Leonie. She feels the full depth and significance of the scene. When she approaches, against all the principles of emergency care, she begins by hugging the children. Intuition overrules training. The neighbour briefs the assembled GP, paramedic and Leonie.

'This couple are renting the lodge. Jill was showing them over and she had a sudden, violent headache and lost consciousness.'

The helicopter paramedic and his crew are there, and with methodical, practised movements, the paramedic is already preparing to establish an airway as he listens. Leonie is able to contribute details of Jill's family and personal medical history where needed, along with descriptions of the resources available on the island, the names and phone numbers of people who may be of assistance. The GP—who is very experienced—offers her medical opinion, too. It is the kind of impromptu team that assembles at all emergencies, where complementary skillsets mesh and clinical responsibility is shared. We agree that we suspect that Jill has suffered a sub-arachnoid haemorrhage.

A basic airway is established, and the paramedic attaches equipment to monitor Jill's respiration and circulation. It is clear Jill is in serious trouble. Leonie hands over the items of equipment—the endotracheal tube, the Cobbs connector, the Ambu bag and angiocaths—and writes down details as information is relayed to her.

Ten minutes have passed since the attempt to resuscitate Jill began.

'I told Mum she should come and see you about her headaches,' her daughter says quietly. 'I was worried about them.'

It turns out that Jill had been suffering from intense headaches in the weeks before this collapse. Typically stoical and fit and healthy, she had dismissed these. Leonie can just hear her laying aside the suggestion that a sore head was serious enough to bother her about.

The conviction is growing among the team that the tentative diagnosis of SAH—sub-arachnoid haemorrhage, or bleed into the arachnoid space, a void beneath one of the delicate membranes covering the brain—is correct. This is usually due to an aneurysm, an abnormality of a blood vessel, and occasionally the catastrophic rupture of an aneurysm is preceded by 'sentinel' headaches, pain caused by lesser bleeds that can serve as warnings if treated as such.

Twenty minutes have passed. The paramedic is satisfied that Jill is sufficiently stable to load aboard the helicopter and evacuate to the Intensive Care Unit at Auckland Hospital. Leonie stands with the two children as the stretcher is wheeled across the grass to the helicopter, the aircraft and the shining chrome and stainless steel of the stretcher glittering in the sun.

The engine note of the helicopter rises and changes as the pilot alters pitch, and with a clattering roar it lifts into the air and swings out towards the bush-clad headland. Soon the sound has faded to a thrum, and the habitual silence of Allom Bay, overlaid with birdsong and cicadas, is restored. There is an emptiness with it, an awful, forlorn sense of aftermath.

The doctor and a neighbour roar off up the track on the quad bike. Leonie sits on the grass with the children as the stranded off-island couple—a pair of middle-aged holidaymakers who would never have believed that their island idyll would start like this—stand bewildered. They have hardly moved all this time.

'Will Mum be OK, Leonie?' Jill's daughter asks.

'We think she is very sick,' she quietly replies. 'They will do everything they can at the hospital. They will want to do special tests to see why your mum's head was hurting so much.'

The children look stricken, but they could see for themselves how desperate their mother's situation was. They are fighting with their tears: like most Barrier children, they have inherited their mother's stoicism.

'I heard you have got some new baby chickens,' Leonie says. 'Do you want to show me?'

Together they wander up the hill, behind the stone house to where the chickens are housed. Away from the others, the children are free to express their fears and, importantly for Leonie too, to cry. They have more questions: Leonie tries to answer frankly. Trying to pretend the situation is otherwise than it is will not help anyone. Leonie also knows that Jill would want her children to be comforted and to be reassured that their dad would be with them as soon as he could arrange it. Leonie the nurse tells them about the medical emergency that their mother has suffered. Leonie, their mother's friend, is there for them, to comfort them. Their father, Jill's partner, is a stonemason by trade, and he is off-island working. Until he can get back, the best and only thing Leonie can do for Jill is to be there for her children in what will be a terrible and confusing time for them.

When they return back down to the guest cottage, after sitting around rather dazed, eventually Jill's other neighbour realises that it is probably best that she scoops the children up and takes them back to her house to await their dad's instructions. The holidaymakers can't decide whether they should stay or return to the mainland. They eventually decide to stay.

During the actual emergency, Leonie kept her own feelings in check. It is not until she gets home and begins to tell Ivan what has happened that she is swamped by grief for her friend and for her friend's children. She weeps again and again over the next 24 hours, especially when news reaches the island that imaging has confirmed an inaccessible SAH that continues to bleed. Jill's life support is turned off 24 hours later, and in a few quiet minutes a wonderful woman, daughter, mother, partner and friend slips from the lives of those who love her like a boat quietly leaving harbour.

Chapter 13

TE PŌ, TE AO

Anyone who grows to be middle-aged learns about the circularities of life, of the cycle by which life renews itself independently of those who are alive. We all see the stars revolve above us, the moon and the sun chase each other across the skies. On an island, you are acutely aware of the tides, and of the seasons—winter brings storms, and it is a time for staying close to home and venturing out only as needed. The raucous call of kākā and the boisterous melody of tūī brawling over territory herald the approach of spring. Summer on Aotea is cicadas and the blaze of pōhutukawa bloom, the annual influx of holidaymakers, long, hot days when the glare of the sand on the east coast can just about blind you. Vegetable gardens are in full production—if you can keep them watered—and the shortcomings of your power and hot water generation arrangements aren't so critical, because of the long twilights and the heat. In autumn, we get our lives back, with the madness of peak season easing. The days are still warm but the nights are cool. As a consolation, the boughs of fruit trees hang low. And then, usually with that first decent storm, we are back into winter.

As a nurse in a rural community, especially on an island, your sense of the cycle is heightened. People are born, they thrive and they die, and you are often standing among the family of those who are birthing, who are celebrating some milestone in life, who are dying or being laid to rest. You are part of it, and you are apart. Sometimes, you might almost imagine you are immune—but of course, you are not.

Back in the days when New Zealanders got about their country in watercraft, drowning was known as 'the New Zealand death'. But with the construction of roads, and the perfection of air travel, for most of us, drowning has become a hazard associated with recreation or freak natural disaster. It is not quite so on Aotea, where people still rely heavily on boats to get to and from their homes and places of work—if their boat is not actually their home, or their place of work. Some of the old families lost people to drowning, or have stories of near misses as they went about their activities on the water. Some of the bays around Great Barrier Island's coast are named for ships that were wrecked there—Cecilia Sudden Bay, Rosalie Bay, Schooner Bay—and there are two celebrity shipwrecks (the SS *Wiltshire* in 1922 and the SS *Wairarapa* in 1894, with the loss of over 120 lives, one of the worst civilian maritime disasters in New Zealand history) that lie mouldering on the seabed. There are five graveyards around the northern part of Aotea where lie many of the *Wairarapa*'s dead. One of the larger ones at Katherine Bay commemorates not only the disaster but also the heroism of the tangata whenua, who saved many lives and cared for the shocked survivors in the aftermath.

During one of Ivan's wanderings along Kaitoke Beach, he found a plastic container with a note scribbled on the back of a cheque book inside. The message, addressed to the writer's children, stated the name of a yacht and promised them that the skipper—the writer—was not afraid to die. Ivan handed the item over to the island's policeman, and he passed it on to his superiors on the mainland. The Police enlisted the Department of Scientific and Industrial Research (DSIR) to conduct tests, and meanwhile conducted enquiries of their own. The DSIR concluded that the item did indeed seem to have been in the water for some considerable time around the same time that the Police established that a yacht of the name mentioned in the message was indeed missing in the Pacific. The yacht was never found.

At last, thinks Adele, as she hears the distinctive note of the *MV Manui*'s engines. A short time later, her navigation lights heave in view as she cruises down the harbour, outward bound for Coromandel.

Adele checks her watch. It is ten o'clock.

Darkness was already falling as Shannon went off grumbling to help Bruno, his business partner, load the mussels from the barge to the *Manui*. The *Manui* was late coming to collect the day's mussel harvest from Shannon's and Bruno's barge, because it had engine trouble. Normally it would have been and gone by three in the afternoon.

Adele gets on with her evening, but by eleven, she is starting to get grumpy herself. Shannon and Bruno are doubtless having a beer and a yarn out on the barge. But as still more time goes by, worry starts seeping past the anger. It reaches the point where she gets in the car and drives to the vantages from which the barge can be seen in the distance. There are no lights on.

Worry is beginning to give way to panic. At home, Adele sits on the bed and forces herself to think what to do. With shaking hands, she picks up the phone and calls Bruno's house.

'You're up late, Adele,' Bruno's wife, Sue, says.

'Is Bruno home?' Adele asks.

'Yes, he's right here, tucked up in bed.'

Adele struggles to get her words out. 'Shannon's not,' she says.

There is a muffled exchange at the end of the line.

'Bruno's getting dressed. He'll go looking.'

After Adele hangs up, she drives down to the wharf to wait. Shannon's aluminium dinghy isn't there, but she already knew it would not be. It seems like an age before she hears an outboard coming towards the wharf, and sees the phosphorescence flashing at the bow of Bruno's boat. It is too dark to tell how many people are aboard until it is practically alongside. With a surge of relief, she sees Shannon sitting next to Bruno.

He is wet and cold—probably hypothermic—but he is alive. He is alive, and Adele waits until he is home and warm and dry before she asks him what happened.

'I got hit by a wave on my way back from the barge,' he says, and names a stretch of water en route that is exposed to the ocean swell from the entrance. 'It tipped me over, and I couldn't get the boat back upright again. So I was just hanging on. After a while, I decided to swim ashore, but I only went a little way before I realised it was a bad idea, especially with my gumboots on. I was lucky I found the boat again. And I was lucky the wind and the tide were with me. I worked out after a while if I hung on, I would wash up eventually. I ended up getting ashore a few bays around. I was pretty happy about it, I can tell you.'

'I was terrified,' Adele says. 'I thought I'd lost you.'

'I saw you!' Shannon says. 'I saw you driving up and down the road. But there's no way up the cliff from the bay, so I couldn't get to you. I was lucky Bruno came along. I had my torch, but I was lucky he saw me. It's nearly out of batteries.'

Bruno lives in a bay with no road access, so he knows the harbour like the back of his hand. He took stock of the wind and tide and worked out where he thought Shannon would wash up if he had found himself in the water. His instincts were correct: in the second bay he checked, he saw the dim light of Shannon's torch waving at him from the stony shore.

Adele refrains from telling Shannon off for not wearing a lifejacket (he draws his own conclusions: after this episode, he always wears one). But she cannot help asking why he kept his heavy gumboots on, especially when he decided he was going to try to swim ashore.

'You must have been hypothermic when you made that decision!' she says.

'No, I figured I would have to walk quite a long way over rocks when I got ashore. Didn't want to hurt my feet. I was lucky.'

Lucky, all right. Lucky, lucky, lucky.

In July 2000, Adele believes her luck has run out.

She is in the bathroom, sobs shaking her shoulders. She started crying silently in bed but did not want to wake Shannon, so here she is in the bathroom surrendering to the emotion.

A mammogram performed over on the mainland confirmed that the lump she had found in her breast was indeed suspicious, so she underwent a biopsy. The results were phoned through just this afternoon. It is malignant, and she has been booked in for a wide local excision (cutting the lump out), along with lymph node dissection (where the lymph nodes that drain the area are taken out and investigated for any sign that the cancer may have spread) and it is then proposed to offer her chemotherapy and radiation.

When she took the surgeon's call, Adele was mostly numb with shock. But the numbness wore off as sleep eluded her, and was replaced with self-pity. She sits in the bathroom and wallows in it for a while. She is not even 50, and yet she might die. A new round of sobbing wracks her.

She has often told her patients that there is sometimes nothing like a good cry. After a while, the surge of emotion has rolled over and past her, and she feels calmer. From the moment we are born, she reflects, we have a finite period of time on Earth.

Do you have any regrets? she asks herself. *What would you change?*

No, she answers. *Nothing.*

Right then. It is off to war we go.

That is how she will treat it.

There are four tactics in the battle against the rogue cells in her body, best summed up as cut, burn, poison and starve. First, the tumour in her breast will be cut out, along with a margin of healthy tissue, in an effort to ensure that all of the cancerous tissue is removed. Then the area is subjected to radiotherapy (burned): cancer cells reproduce at a faster rate than normal cells, and fast-growing cells are more susceptible to radiation damage. At the completion of the course of radiotherapy, everyone can be reasonably confident the local area is free of disease. But to make sure of it, and also to target any cells that may have metastasised (spread) beyond the primary site, a range of highly toxic drugs are administered, once again to target fast-growing cells. Once chemotherapy is complete, the disease can be considered to have been eradicated. But because Adele's particular cancer is enhanced by one of the hormones that naturally occur in her body, drugs to alter the hormonal cell wall to deprive any remaining cancer cells of the ability to utilise that hormone are offered. In effect, any remaining rogue cells are starved.

All of this will be pretty rugged. Because they target fast-growing cells, the radiation and the chemotherapy also affect some normal tissues that are also fast-growing, such as the linings of the mouth and gut and, of course, hair follicles (although, as it turns out, Adele is fortunate and does not lose her hair). The chemotherapy drugs have a range of side-effects: which ones she will suffer, and how severe they will be, is unpredictable, as it all depends on the individual. And quite apart from the routine demands of this regime, it will be made all the harder for Adele, of course, because she will have to travel to the mainland for each step of the process.

But as it always does, the island community draws around Adele as news spreads. A friend of the family tosses her an envelope in which there is a heavy object.

'What's this?' she asks.

'Keys to our place in Auckland,' he says. 'You'll be needing somewhere to stay over there. And the car key's there, too. Pretty hard getting around Auckland without a car.'

This is typical of the kind of support she gets. And when she wakes after her surgery, she finds her hospital bed surrounded by vases of flowers. A nurse brings in a big cardboard box full of get-well cards from the children of Kaitoke School.

The treatment regime is manageable, Adele does not focus on it: the side-effect of not undergoing it, as she explains to people who commiserate with her, is potentially death, so anything short of that is fine. People—professionals and well-meaning amateurs alike—give her articles on special cancer diets and foods to avoid at all costs. She should not eat sugar or dairy. She should avoid coffee—or drinking it, anyway: coffee enemas are in vogue. But Adele has seen too many people succumb to cancer while enduring coffee enemas and trying to live on beetroot juice. If she is going to die, she reasons, then she will do it enjoying all of the foods that she loves.

During the treatment period, Adele takes six months off work and focuses on recovery. She feels her strength returning. Soon she finds herself forgetting about cancer. After a year or two, she hardly gives it a thought. And, ten years on, she celebrates. She has won the battle. That particular cancer will not kill her.

Sometimes you feel that life on the island is just too hard. But the trips to Auckland, such as Adele's trips for treatment, and the struggle there with traffic and the relentlessly fast pace remind us how fortunate we actually are. On Aotea, we can drive for 40 minutes along a road overhung by mānuka and ponga without seeing another vehicle. Each corner opens a new vista of mountain and bush and white sand, and a different perspective on the ocean and the horizon, the sea and the cloudscape. If you do pass another vehicle, the driver will lift a finger from the steering wheel as you lift yours. In the city, you notice how few people you know: on the island, you notice the strangers, and in winter there are few.

And life has got easier. The advent first of the Community Health Trust, then of Aotea Health, has blessed us with the resources that we lacked in the early days. We have access to equipment and people, and as a consequence we have a modicum of that thing that was the scarcest commodity when we started: time for ourselves and our families. We still work full-time, but we are not so constantly on-call, and nor do we live in such a fishbowl as we used to.

Our lives have changed, as the cycle of which we are a part has creaked around, as it inevitably does. Leonie and Ivan's children have grown. Alastair was still a teenager when their younger two were born, and he is well established in his medical career these days. First Amiria, then Jordan, reached the age where the island no longer had the educational resources for them. It is traditional at this point for Barrier families to choose where their children will seek secondary schooling. The Howies had already arranged their option: to attend a public boarding school, and one by one, Leonie and Ivan packed their children off. It was a culture shock for both of them. There had been few choices open for Amiria's secondary education: of the public schools that still offered full board, St Mary's had closed, leaving Epsom Girls' Grammar, which her aunts and cousins had attended. But she quickly found her feet there, thriving among the opportunities that a big school had to offer her to make friends and play sport. Jordan's choice was probably made when he was still a baby, his dad being an old boy of Auckland Grammar School—every time they travelled past, Ivan would point it out, saying: 'There's Jordan's school.' Jordan suffered terribly from home-sickness at first—the regimentation, the uniform, the big city, the sheer number of other people were bound to deliver a culture shock—but we breed them tough on Aotea. Leonie and Ivan gave him the option during the worst times to return to the island but he stuck it out, and after the initial adjustment, he, too, began to thrive. Both are well along their own journeys now. Jordan is an engineering geologist, and Amiria followed down the medicine pathway. The Barrier has offered her its own, distinctive experiences. During her holidays through medical school she worked as a receptionist at the Health Centre. The locals soon cottoned on to the fact she was training to be a doctor, and rather than bother the qualified staff beyond the reception desk, they began consulting the receptionist on their ailments.

'Look,' one said, hitching up his shorts as Amiria hastily averted her eyes. 'Know what this is?' Amiria shuddered to think. 'You'll see a few of these. It's a hernia scar.'

They viewed all this as part of her learning and wanted to help 'educate' her.

It took Shannon some time to discover the trick of standing upright on Aotea, but once he did, there was no shifting him. He retired in 2013, after 21 years as a mussel farmer and even longer as a resident of the Barrier and chief support to the Public Health Nurse, Northern Riding. And at the time of writing, Dr Ivan Howie is retiring too, after more than 36 years of service as a GP on Aotea, for many of them *the* GP on Aotea.

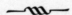

Adele has won the battle, but not, as it turns out, the war. A few years after her original diagnosis, one of Adele's beautiful younger sisters developed ovarian cancer. From the outset, the prognosis was poor, but she managed to battle the disease for seven years, showing her family and friends how to be brave and strong every step along her very sad journey. Apart from when she first moved to the island, it was during this period that Adele felt the isolation of her life on Great Barrier more acutely than at any other time. Spending time with her family on the mainland meant finding a window among her midwifery obligations to the pregnant women on the island and finding cover for her nursing post, not to mention the disruption that had to be allowed for the operation of the mussel farm when the need to go away fell during the busy time. Then there was the erratic schedule of ferry and air services to reckon with. You cannot just spontaneously leave the island. As she was in the air heading to Auckland, her sister passed away. She left Adele and her three remaining sisters and brother with four amazing nieces as a constant reminder of what a wonderful mother, wife and sibling she had been.

As part of the diagnosis of her disease, Adele's sister also underwent genetic testing, and it was found that the family carries the BRCA2 gene mutation. This means Adele and two of her three surviving sisters who have the mutation have a fifty to eighty per cent lifetime risk of developing breast cancer and a twenty to forty per cent risk of developing ovarian cancer. This elevated the chances of Adele developing cancer in her unaffected breast to thirty to fifty per cent.

She was considering prophylactic mastectomies—the complete removal of the tissue of both breasts as a precautionary measure— when she discovered a cancerous lump in her right breast, which had been previously unaffected. There is some research to show that cancers of the right breast are more aggressive than those in the left: regardless of whether this is true or not, this round of the disease is more aggressive than Adele's first. But if the disease is more determined, so is she. There is no wailing or grieving this time. Instead, she is thankful that her tumour is in a place that was easier to detect early, whereas her sister's hadn't been. There are times when the treatment is like a ghastly step back in time, but Adele sees it through. She wins the second great battle for her life, but it is too early to declare the war to be over. It is now a waiting game. But then again, it is a waiting game for all of us, in the end.

EPILOGUE

The speeches are over. We have said our farewells to Jill, whom we have known as a patient, mother, daughter, partner, grandmother and, above all, friend. Others have known her, too, in many different ways, and each has their little fragment of the whole to show. The work of the gathering has been to stitch these together into a single whole, and as we leave we reflect on how well it has been done. It is something we can draw around ourselves when we remember her, this shared yet particoloured experience.

There was only one Jill, but there are many Jills: we know these people, the islanders, the Barrierites, on lots of levels, just as we know Aotea itself, through the intimate tread of our feet on narrow clay paths through the bush, or the business-like rumble of tyres on the gravel of the road, or the glorious panorama it makes from the high points, or from the air. We know the heat of the summer and the burn of the sun, the smell of mānuka and road dust, the rank smell of the raupō swamps and the tang of salt. We know the cold sting of the surf and of rainwater in the shower, and the raw bite of a winter sou'wester. There are the hard times, and there are the good times: we can remember all of them, and they have shaped who we are.

Adele reflects on her first meeting with Jill's father, and then her first meeting with Jill. She thinks about the raw clearing that she chanced upon on one of her early visiting rounds, and the man who would become Jill's partner and the father of her younger children. She thinks about the house that was built there, and the other families she has visited where successive babies have marked stages in their progress: from rough shelter, to simple house, to something more substantial, to something well and truly comfortable.

Leonie remembers Jill as she first met her, the very picture of the Barrier woman, staunch and practical and warm and hospitable. She aged as Leonie herself has aged, but it was the way of things that they would not grow old together, as Leonie had supposed they would. She feels her loss keenly, but she is also conscious of how lucky she is to have known Jill, to have shared her journey (even its bitter end) and to have known others in the same way.

This is what it is to be a nurse in a place like Aotea. You do not clock into the job and then clock out of it. It enfolds you, as the arms of Allom Bay enfold us now. It defines you, and it gives to you even as it takes away from you. You can walk away from it, just as we walk sadly up the clay track away from Jill and the stories that we shared with her. But it follows you, like memory. It is with you, always.

Acknowledgements

We gratefully acknowledge those islanders who have granted us permission to tell their personal stories and those who assisted us in validating the historical data included in the book. Without these people, there could not have been a book.

Our grateful thanks to our island-based colleagues (past and present)—we thank you for being part of 'Team Aotea Health' and for your service to the island community.

To Dr Jean Ross, who led us on a rural-nursing academic journey— we hope that this book has done justice to and adds knowledge of the characteristics of rural people, their communities and the nurses who care for them.

Our thanks also to Jenny Hellen and her team at Allen & Unwin, who encouragingly and tactfully nurtured us. To John McCrystal for his sensitive editing of the stories and for so capably dealing with the challenge of combining two voices in one book.

To our families—and especially our very tolerant husbands—who have provided unconditional support in the work that we do and over the years that we have lived and breathed this work.

To Dr Ivan Howie, who shared our vision of a health service specially tailored to the islanders' needs, and who has been a teacher, mentor and friend by helping us both to fly in our professional roles.

Finally, we would like to pay tribute to our mothers, who are no longer with us. By example, they shaped us into the women we have become and pointed us along the nursing and midwifery pathway that we have never had cause to regret.

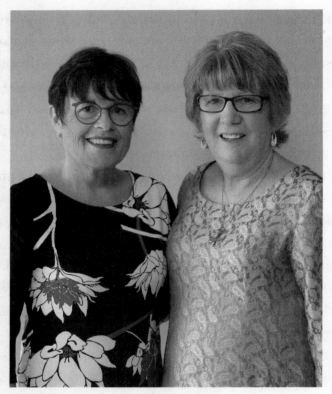
Leonie Howie (left) and Adele Robertson.

About the authors

Adele Robertson and Leonie Howie are rural nurse specialists and midwives on Great Barrier Island Aotea. They both hold Masters of Nursing degrees and, along with Dr Ivan Howie, are cofounders and directors of the island's primary health service, Aotea Health. They have been fortunate to live and work on Great Barrier Island for more than 30 years—a beautiful place that is, as the islanders call it, a world of its own.

This book is their attempt to share the uniqueness of the place and the people, and to show the challenges and complexity of what it means to work in such a remote rural environment. Adele and Leonie belong to a community of hardy and rugged individuals who are used to coping with adversity and are never afraid to pitch in and offer support. As the two nurses have learned during their time on Aotea, the islanders are infinitely capable in both their outlook and their ability to care for each other.

This book has only been made possible by the individuals and families who have allowed Leonie and Adele to tell their stories— stories of struggle, stories of sorrow, stories of celebration. Adele and Leonie's stories are the islanders' stories; they are all woven together. As 'insiders', Adele and Leonie do not notice what people wear, how they look or what their employment is; instead, they celebrate the resilience, resourcefulness and caring spirit of the locals, and share a pride in the island of Aotea. They know, and are blessed to be part of, a community in which people care about each other.

Want ideas for what to read next, competitions and news about your favourite authors?

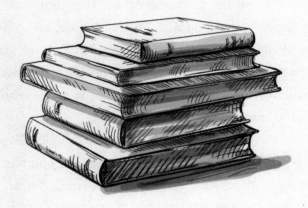

Join us at:

Facebook
www.facebook.com/AllenAndUnwinNZ

Instagram
www.instagram.com/AllenAndUnwinNZ

Twitter
www.twitter.com/AllenAndUnwinNZ

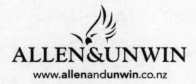